FREE Study Skills DVD Offer

Dear Customer,

Thank you for your purchase from Mometrix! We consider it an honor and privilege that you have purchased our product and want to ensure your satisfaction.

As a way of showing our appreciation and to help us better serve you, we have developed a Study Skills DVD that we would like to give you for <u>FREE</u>. **This DVD covers our "best practices" for studying for your exam, from how to use our study materials to how to prepare for the day of the test.**

All that we ask is that you email us your feedback that would describe your experience so far with our product. Good, bad or indifferent, we want to know what you think!

To get your **FREE Study Skills DVD**, email <u>freedvd@mometrix.com</u> with "FREE STUDY SKILLS DVD" in the subject line and the following information in the body of the email:

    a. The name of the product you purchased.

    b. Your product rating on a scale of 1-5, with 5 being the highest rating.

    c. Your feedback. It can be long, short, or anything in-between, just your impressions and experience so far with our product. Good feedback might include how our study material met your needs and will highlight features of the product that you found helpful.

    d. Your full name and shipping address where you would like us to send your free DVD.

If you have any questions or concerns, please don't hesitate to contact me directly.

Thanks again!

Sincerely,

Jay Willis
Vice President of Sales
<u>jay.willis@mometrix.com</u>
1-800-673-8175

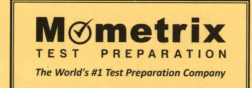

TABLE OF CONTENTS

Top 20 Test Taking Tips 4
Physical Care Skills 5
    Activities of Daily Living 5
    Basic Nursing Skills 9
    Restorative Skills 42
Psychosocial Care Skills 49
Role of the Nurse Aide 59
Practice Test 83
    Practice Questions 83
    Answers and Explanations 94
Secret Key #1 - Time is Your Greatest Enemy 104
    Pace Yourself 104
Secret Key #2 - Guessing is not Guesswork 104
    Monkeys Take the Test 104
    $5 Challenge 105
Secret Key #3 - Practice Smarter, Not Harder 106
    Success Strategy 106
Secret Key #4 - Prepare, Don't Procrastinate 106
Secret Key #5 - Test Yourself 107
General Strategies 107
Special Report: What Your Test Score Will Tell You About Your IQ 113
Special Report: How to Overcome Test Anxiety 115
    Lack of Preparation 115
    Physical Signals 116
    Nervousness 116
    Study Steps 118
    Helpful Techniques 119
Special Report: Retaking the Test: What Are Your Chances at Improving Your Score? 124
Special Report: Additional Bonus Material 126

Top 20 Test Taking Tips

1. Carefully follow all the test registration procedures
2. Know the test directions, duration, topics, question types, how many questions
3. Setup a flexible study schedule at least 3-4 weeks before test day
4. Study during the time of day you are most alert, relaxed, and stress free
5. Maximize your learning style; visual learner use visual study aids, auditory learner use auditory study aids
6. Focus on your weakest knowledge base
7. Find a study partner to review with and help clarify questions
8. Practice, practice, practice
9. Get a good night's sleep; don't try to cram the night before the test
10. Eat a well balanced meal
11. Know the exact physical location of the testing site; drive the route to the site prior to test day
12. Bring a set of ear plugs; the testing center could be noisy
13. Wear comfortable, loose fitting, layered clothing to the testing center; prepare for it to be either cold or hot during the test
14. Bring at least 2 current forms of ID to the testing center
15. Arrive to the test early; be prepared to wait and be patient
16. Eliminate the obviously wrong answer choices, then guess the first remaining choice
17. Pace yourself; don't rush, but keep working and move on if you get stuck
18. Maintain a positive attitude even if the test is going poorly
19. Keep your first answer unless you are positive it is wrong
20. Check your work, don't make a careless mistake

Physical Care Skills

Activities of Daily Living

Activities of daily living (ADLs) are tasks that are required to keep a person healthy and functional. Often, a person's level of health is determined by his ability to perform ADLs. The tasks are divided into two subgroups: basic ADLs and instrumental ADLs.

- Basic ADLs are tasks people must be perform in order to care for themselves. These include bathing, dressing, feeding, toileting, and walking.
- Instrumental ADLs are tasks performed in order to live independently within the community. These include shopping, cooking, housework, medication management, and money management.

Hygiene

The components of hygiene are the tasks that are necessary to promote patient health through cleanliness. These tasks include hair care, nail care, mouth care, bathing, and dressing. Hair care includes a gentle brushing and inspection of the patient's scalp. Nail care involves keeping the patient's nails trimmed and inspecting the patient's nail beds. Mouth care is performed to prevent tooth decay and to examine the patient's oral mucosa for sores or signs of infection. Bathing is done to keep the patient's skin clean and to inspect for lesions; this includes perineal care. The nursing assistant must also ensure that dependent patients are able to dress and undress themselves properly.

<u>Purposes of a bath</u>

Over time, irritants can build on the patient's skin, which can cause a rash or skin breakdown. These irritants can also cause itching, which may provoke the patient to scratch the skin, creating a source of infection. Bathing cleanses the patient's skin of these irritants. Bathing can also promote patient relaxation and increase circulation. Bathing presents an opportunity to perform a thorough assessment of the patient's skin. Any signs of breakdown or lesions should be immediately reported. Furthermore, the patient's skin should be closely monitored for dryness, as this can cause cracking of the patient's skin.

- A tub bath is preferred when the patient is strong enough to get into and out of the bathtub. It involves completely washing the patient, including performing perineal care. A tub bath can be given daily. However, if the patient's skin is showing signs of dryness, the frequency may be reduced to two or three times a week.
- A bed bath is given to a patient when he is unable to ambulate. A complete bed bath involves cleansing the patient's skin and changing the patient's linens.
- If the patient is incontinent of urine or stool, a partial bath may be given. This involves cleansing only those parts of the body that have been soiled and changing only those linens that are dirty.

Equipment to perform a bed bath: A bed bath can be a time-consuming procedure, depending upon the patient's level of activity. One way to facilitate a bed bath is to make sure that all of the necessary supplies are present prior to starting the bath.

- A nurse aide will require a basin of water, soap, and lotion.

- The water should be warmed to between 105 and 115 degrees.
- The nurse aide will need several washcloths and at least two towels.
- The nurse aide must also have a pair of gloves to wear while giving the bath.

Linens should be changed while the bed bath is being performed. In order to change the bed, the nurse aide will need a fitted sheet, a bed pad, a flat sheet, a blanket, and pillowcases.

A.M. and H.S. care

A.M. care is typically done in the morning, prior to any scheduled medical procedures. A.M. care involves a complete bath, shaving, dressing, hair care, oral care, and nails care, and may require changing of the bed linens.

Hour of sleep (H.S.) care is done at bedtime. H.S. care involves an abbreviated form of skin care, including washing the patient's face and hands. Oral care should also be performed. A back rub may be given for 5 to 10 minutes to ensure the patient is relaxed and ready for sleep. Additional tasks may be performed, depending upon the patient's level of health and activity.

Hair care

Hair care is a procedure that helps to improve patient comfort and morale. It stimulates blood circulation within the scalp. Hair washing also removes excess oils and bacteria. Frequency of hair care depends upon the amount of oil that has accumulated in the patient's hair, as well as the level of dryness of the scalp.

- The nurse aide must be vigilant while performing hair care.
- Head lice, an excessive amount of dandruff, or sores on the scalp should be reported to the nurse immediately if noticed by the nurse aide. Such findings may

require special precautions to be taken while performing hair care in the future.

Patient's nails

A nurse aide should exercise caution when providing nail care to patients who are receiving anticoagulation therapy as this type of medication puts the patient at an increased risk for bleeding.

- Nail care should not be performed on patients with a history of diabetes or decreased circulation in their feet.
- Diabetes and low circulation affect the ability of the tissue to repair itself. As a result, even the smallest cut on the skin places the patient at risk for severe ulcers on the feet.
- Prior to performing nail care; the nurse aide should check the facility policies to ensure that nail cutting falls within her scope of practice.

Importance of nail care: Nail care is important for a number of reasons. The primary purpose of nail care is to remove bacteria and dirt from the patient's nail beds, preventing the spread of microorganisms.

- Appropriate nail care also ensures the patient's nails are not sharp or jagged, which increases the risk of infection from breakage of the skin.
- While performing nail care, the nursing assistant has the opportunity to inspect the patient's nail beds for any signs of inflammation or fungal growth.
- Any signs of infection or discoloration should immediately be reported to the nurse.

Four stages of pressure sores

Pressure sores are divided into four stages, classified by the depth of the wound.

- Stage I pressure sore refers to an area of redness that is typically located over a bony prominence. The reddened area may feel painful or warm to the touch.
- Stage II pressure sore refers to wearing away of the first layer of skin, revealing a pink wound bed below.
- Stage III pressure sore extends past the full thickness of the skin; fatty tissue may be visualized. Tunneling may also be present.
- Stage IV pressure sore is the most severe, referring to a loss of enough skin tissue to reveal muscle tissue or bone.

<u>Procedures to prevent skin irritation</u>
Skin irritation can result in sores and infection. There are a number of measures a nurse aide can take to prevent skin irritation from occurring.

- One way to avoid skin rash or irritation is to completely cleanse the skin of any urine or feces if the patient has soiled himself. Because urine and stool is acidic in nature, skin breakdown can occur quickly if left close to the patient's skin. If the patient is incontinent, applying water resistant lotion will protect the skin by creating a barrier that will prevent rashes or breakdown.
- Frequent repositioning should also be performed to prevent skin breakdown. A bedridden patient should be turned every two hours to prevent breakdown over bony prominences.

Oral care

Performing oral care presents an ideal opportunity to examine the patient's oral mucosa for abnormalities.

- The nurse aide should carefully observe the patient's mouth for any sores, redness, or bleeding on the patient's lips or gums.
- Cracking may occur on the patient's lips as a result of dryness.
- The nurse aide should also be observant for any odor that may occur as a result of infection.
- Thrush is a fungal infection that can develop as a result of poor oral care or after taking certain medications. If thrush is present, the patient may appear with white patches covering the tongue or gums. The patient may also complain of a thick, furry feeling in the mouth.

Dressing a dependent patient

When the patient has suffered a stroke, it can result in weakness on one side of the patient's body. Often, the patient may require assistance in daily activities, such as dressing.

- It is important to teach the patient how to clothe himself safely to promote independence and decrease the risk of falling.
- Before beginning to assist the patient in undressing, make sure the clean set of clothes is within easy reach.
- When putting on clothing, the patient should be taught to dress the weakened side first. For example, a patient with weakness on the right side should insert the right arm into the sleeve first.
- When undressing, the patient should be taught to remove clothing from the strong side first.

Measuring intake and output

Intake and output (I&O) is an important indicator of fluid balance.

- Intake is calculated by measuring all of the fluid the patient drinks.
- Output is calculated by measuring all of the fluid the patient secretes, including urine, stool, and emesis.

All measurements should be recorded in cubic centimeters (cc). Calculating I&O over a period of a few days can give an indication of the patient's fluid status. Ideally, intake should equal output. If intake exceeds output, then the patient may be fluid overloaded. If output exceeds intake, the patient may be dehydrated.

Therapeutic diets

The diet that is prescribed for a patient depends upon the individual's health history.

- A regular diet has no dietary restrictions; patients can eat whatever they like.
- A calorie count diet is typically ordered for diabetic patients; it limits the amount of sugar the patient takes in and counts the number of calories and carbohydrates the patient consumes.
- A low-sodium diet is prescribed to limit the amount of salt ingested by patients with a history of renal impairment or hypertension.
- A cardiac diet is ordered for patients with a history of cardiac problems; while on this diet, they are served low-fat, low-calorie, and low-sodium foods.
- NPO (nothing by mouth) is a diet that is ordered for patients who are not allowed to eat. It is typically ordered in anticipation of medical testing or a surgical

procedure. Patient status will also be made NPO if it is unsafe for the individual to eat, such as a patient who is intubated, sedated, or unable to swallow properly.

- A clear liquid diet is the first diet prescribed after a patient is taken off NPO status. It is typically ordered to allow the patient to eat without experiencing nausea.
- A mechanical soft diet is prescribed for patients who have difficulty chewing, such as patients who do not have their dentures. It is also intended to help patients to transition from NPO to a regular diet.

USDA dietary guideline changes

The United States Department of Agriculture began issuing nutrition guidelines in 1894, and in 1943 the department began promoting the Basic 7 food groups. In 1956, Basic 7 was replaced with the Basic Four food groups. These were fruits and vegetables, cereals and breads, milk, and meat. Basic Four lasted until 1992, when it was replaced with the Food Pyramid, which divided food into six groups: 1) Bread, cereal, rice, pasta 2) Fruit 3) Vegetables 4) Meat, poultry, fish, dry beans, eggs, nuts 5) Milk, yogurt, cheese 6) Fats, oils, sweets. The Food Pyramid also provided recommendations for the number of daily servings from each group.

The USDA's Food Pyramid was heavily criticized for being vague and confusing, and in 2011 it was replaced with MyPlate. MyPlate is much easier to understand, as it consists of a picture of a dinner plate divided into four sections, visually illustrating how our daily diet should be distributed among the various food groups. Vegetables and grains each take up 30% of the plate, while fruits and proteins each constitute 20% of the plate. There is also a representation of a cup, marked Dairy, alongside the plate. The idea behind MyPlate is that it's much easier for people to grasp the idea that half of a meal should consist of fruits and vegetables than it is for them to understand serving sizes for all the different kinds of foods they eat on a regular basis.

Different types of nutrients and their importance: Nutrients are elements in nature that are necessary in order to live. Our bodies absorb the nutrients from the foods we eat. Nutrients are divided into six groups: carbohydrates, proteins, fats, minerals, vitamins, and water.

- Carbohydrates are composed primarily of sugar and serve as the main source of energy.
- Protein is made primarily of amino acids and aids in tissue repair.
- Fats are composed of fatty acids and are essential for cell membrane integrity and thermal regulation.
- Minerals and vitamins are needed to aid metabolism and a number of other body processes.
- Water acts as a solvent and is also required for a number of body processes.

Promotion of hydration: Water is a vitally important nutrient. It aids in metabolism, temperature regulation, and elimination of body waste. Water is constantly lost through normal sweating, elimination, and exhalation. Certain states, such as illness and increased activity, can cause increased water loss.

- It is recommended that the patient take in at least 1500cc to 2000cc or 8 to 10 glasses of water every day to maintain hydration and replace lost body fluids.
- If the patient does not receive an adequate amount of fluids, dehydration may occur. If left uncorrected, dehydration can be a fatal condition.

When it is important to assist in feeding
The amount of feeding assistance that should be provided depends upon the individual patient. Some patients will not require assistance to feed themselves.

- If the patient is able to feed himself, he should be allowed to do so to encourage independence.
- Some assistance may be required, such as cutting larger portions and opening beverages.
- Some patients, such as those who suffer from blindness, may only need verbal cues to eat.
- Some patients are unable to feed themselves as a result of weakness or paralysis of the upper body. These patients will require their food be cut and each bite fed to them.
- Nurse aides should be careful to take their time and not rush the feeding.
- Aides should ensure the patient has chewed and swallowed every bite, before offering the next bit of food.

Basic Nursing Skills

Infection Control

Hand washing

Microorganisms are present on all surfaces and can be transferred via touch. Certain microorganisms can cause illness or infection if they come into contact with a person whose immune system has been compromised. As a result, hand washing is a vital part of infection control. If properly done, hand washing removes visible dirt and germs from the hands. It prevents transmission of germs from the nurse aide to the patient or from one patient to another patient. Warm water, antimicrobial soap, and firm friction applied to all areas of the hand while washing are all key factors in ensuring that the hands are clean and free of germs.

Hand washing
- Before beginning to wash, remove any jewelry on your hands.
- Run the water until it is warm, and then wet hands to the wrist.
- Apply a small amount of soap.
- Continue to work the soap into lather for at least 30 seconds, using firm friction between the fingers, underneath the fingernails, and up the wrists.
- Make sure to keep your hands lower than the elbows to prevent germs from traveling up the arm.
- If your hands have been soiled with body fluids, hand washing should be performed for at least one minute.
- Rinse hands thoroughly with warm water, and then dry your hands.
- When your hands are dry, use part of the towel to turn the faucet off.

Hand washing should be performed: frequently to prevent transmission of germs.
- The nurse aide should wash her hands prior to eating, after going to the bathroom, or after sneezing.
- The aide should also wash her hands prior to feeding the patient, before performing any procedures with the patient and after the procedure is complete.
- Hand washing should be performed after coming into contact with a patient's wound, with soiled linen, or with any patient body fluids, even if the nurse aide was wearing gloves at the time.
- The nurse aide should also wash her hands prior to leaving the patient's room.

Proper hand washing is the key to infection control. Because germs run off the hands while hand washing is performed, it is important to ensure that hands do not touch the inside of the sink while washing.
- If a nurse aide's hands touch the inside of the sink, then hand washing should be repeated to ensure her hands have not become contaminated.

Washing with bar soap: A wet surface of bar soap can provide a medium for germs to grow.
- Prior to beginning to wash hands, rub the soap vigorously to remove the outermost layer of soap.
- Then, once hand washing has been completed, rinse the soap with warm water.

Cleansing hands with alcohol scrub: hand sanitizers have been approved as an adjunct to hand washing in the health care setting. They work by removing the outer layer of oils on the hand, killing any bacteria on the hand in the process.
- To use alcohol scrub, take a dime-sized amount into your dominant hand.
- Rub your hands together vigorously for at least thirty seconds.
- Make sure to rub between your fingers, between your knuckles, and beneath the fingernails.
- If, after thirty seconds, your hands are still damp, allow them to air dry.
- Once your hands have dried, they are considered clean.

Alcohol scrub versus hand washing: though hand sanitizer has been approved as an adjunct for hand washing, it was not intended to replace it. There are instances in which hand washing is preferred over use of an alcohol-based hand sanitizer.

- A nurse aide should wash her hands if they have been soiled with secretions.
- Hand washing should be used prior to eating and after using the bathroom.
- Even if hand sanitizer is used, hands should occasionally be washed to remove any residue that can build up as a result of frequent use of alcohol scrub.

Isolation

Isolation refers to special measures taken to prevent the spread of germs. The goal is to protect other patients and hospital staff while providing care to the patient. Isolation may be required if the patient has a particularly infectious disease, such as tuberculosis or Varicella. The patient may also be placed into isolation if he has a drug-resistant bacterium, such as methicillin-resistant staphylococcus aureus (MRSA) or clostridium difficile (C. diff). Depending upon the type of isolation, the nurse aide may be required to wear an isolation gown, gloves, or a mask while providing care for the patient.

Types of isolation
There are three types of isolation.

- Contact precautions are intended to limit the spread of microorganisms that might be transmitted by direct contact with a contaminated surface. If a patient is in contact isolation, he should be in a private room that is clearly marked. When providing care to the patient, the nurse aide should wear an isolation gown and gloves at all times while in the room.
- Droplet precautions are intended to limit the spread of microorganisms that are transmitted via mucous or respiratory secretions. A patient who requires droplet precautions should be placed in a private room. A nurse aide should wear a mask and gloves when caring for a patient who is in droplet precautions.
- Airborne precautions are intended to prevent the spread of airborne microorganisms that can survive for long periods of time in the environment. While on airborne precautions, the patient should be placed in a negative pressure room. While caring for the patient, the nurse aide should wear a mask or respirator and gloves.

Items for a patient in isolation
The nursing assistant should take care to ensure that germs from a patient in isolation are not spread amid the patient population.

- A cart should be placed outside of the patient's room containing isolation equipment that should be donned prior to entering the room.
- This includes waterproof isolation gowns, gloves, and masks, as well as a garbage bag for waste disposal. Germicidal wipes should also be available to clean the equipment that must be shared with the rest of the patient population.
- The patient in isolation can also be provided with disposable equipment that might ordinarily be shared among the patient population, such as single-use

stethoscopes and blood pressure cuffs.

Personal protective equipment (PPE):
Gloves are the most commonly used piece of protective equipment in the health care setting. They are typically made of thin vinyl or nitrile rubber and are intended for single use. They should be used whenever there is a risk of touching infectious material or body fluids.

- Gowns are typically made of thin plastic or synthetic waterproof fibers. They are typically worn over the uniform whenever the patient is in contact isolation.
- Face protection falls into two categories.
  - Facemasks are worn over the nose and mouth to prevent inhalation of infectious material.
  - Goggles are worn over the eyes to prevent introduction of infectious materials to the eyes.

When dealing with a copious amount of secretions, a face shield can be worn in place of a facemask and goggles.

Procedure for putting on an isolation gown, gloves, and mask & removal
Isolation equipment should be donned before entering an isolation room.

- The gown should be unfolded and held with the opening toward your back.
- Place your arms through the sleeves.
- Tie the gown securely behind the neck and at the waist.
- Then, put on the facemask, making sure your nose and mouth are covered.
- Gloves should be applied last and worn so they cover the cuffs of the isolation gown.

Isolation gear should be removed prior to leaving the room.

- The gloves should be removed first.
- Grasp the first glove at the wrist and pull to remove it.
- Then ball the used glove in the hand that is still gloved.
- Grasp the remaining glove at the wrist and pull to remove it.
- Next, remove the gown and the mask.
- Once the gloves, gown, and mask have been removed, wash your hands.

Procedure for removal of soiled linen
Care must be taken while removing soiled linen from an isolation room. Because the linen bag was in the isolation room, it is considered contaminated. The soiled linen bag must be placed inside a clean bag to prevent contamination.

- While the nursing assistant is bathing the patient, soiled linen should be placed in a plastic linen bag.
- Once bathing has been completed, the linen bag should be tied securely shut.
- Another aide standing outside the door should hold a second linen bag open while the first bag is placed inside; the second bag should also be tied securely shut.
- The double-bagged linen bag should be left outside while the nurse aide removes her isolation gown, gloves, and mask, and washes her hands.
- Then, the soiled linen can be taken to the soiled utility room.

Precautions to take to prevent the spread of microorganisms while changing linens:
While removing dirty linens, the nurse aide should wear gloves and avoid holding them close to her body.

- Soiled linens should not be shaken out as this may release germs into the air.
- Once all of the soiled linens have been removed from the bed and put into the appropriate receptacle, the nurse aide should remove her gloves and wash her hands.
- She should then securely tie the linen bag closed and place it in the soiled utility room.
- Clean linens should be carefully unfolded and placed on the bed.
- Any linen that has fallen on the floor should be considered contaminated; it should be placed in the soiled utility bin and replaced with clean linen.

Universal precautions

Universal precautions involve treating all patient secretions as if they contain a pathogen, resulting in the avoidance of direct contact with any secretions. Universal precautions are practiced in the health care setting whenever there is the risk of coming into contact with blood or body fluids. The precautions include wearing gloves when collecting blood or handling anything that may have been contaminated with blood. Use of other protective equipment may be necessary, such as wearing a face shield when suctioning copious secretions or a facemask to protect oneself from airborne secretions. If blood or body fluids have contaminated a work surface, it should be cleaned using the appropriate disinfectant.

- Cleaning refers to the process that removes visible dirt or soiled material from a surface. It typically involves using water or a detergent to rinse the surface. Cleaning must be performed prior to disinfection or sterilization.
- Disinfection is defined as the process that destroys most microorganisms on the surface of a piece of equipment. The disinfectant that is used is typically chemical in nature, though some pieces of equipment may be disinfected using heat.
- Sterilization refers to the process that removes all forms of microbial life from a piece of equipment.

Risk for infection from patient care equipment

The level of risk for infection refers to the likelihood that a piece of equipment will contain infectious pathogens on its surface; it aids in determining the proper level of cleaning prior to subsequent use.

- Low-risk or noncritical items are pieces of equipment that come into contact with intact skin, such as stethoscopes. Noncritical items also include inanimate objects in the environment, such as countertops and walls. These items only require cleaning with a detergent prior to subsequent use.
- Intermediate-risk items are those that come in close contact with mucous membranes but do not penetrate the skin, such as thermometers or respiratory equipment. These items require cleaning with a high-level disinfectant before they are ready for use.
- High-risk items, such as surgical instruments and devices, have penetrated the skin and are at high risk for contamination by microorganisms. These items require sterilization before they are ready for subsequent use.

Steps for cleaning equipment
Cleaning refers to the process of removing dirt or organic material from

the surface of a piece of equipment. If an item is not properly cleaned, subsequent disinfection or sterilization may not be effective.

- Gloves should be worn while cleaning equipment.
- Thoroughly wipe each piece of equipment with a detergent, rubbing with firm pressure to remove any dirt or organic material.
- Once the organic material and dirt has been removed, rinse the surface thoroughly with water and allow it to dry prior to subsequent use.
- Hand washing should be performed after cleaning any equipment.

Steps for sterilizing equipment:
Sterilization requires a piece of equipment be exposed to extreme dry heat or a chemical sterilant to remove all microorganisms. Equipment is typically exposed to dry heat during the autoclaving process. Autoclaving is considered to be the most effective method of sterilization. Chemical sterilization is used for equipment unable to tolerate high temperatures, such as fluids and rubber.

- Care must be taken when handling sterile equipment.
- Any contact with a non-sterile surface will introduce new microorganisms to the equipment. When a piece of sterile equipment is prepared for use, it should be handled using sterile technique.

Infection

Infections are divided into two groups, localized and systemic.

- A localized infection occurs when a virus or bacteria begins to grow in a small area of the body. This can occur in wounds or surgical sites if not treated properly. Signs and symptoms of a localized infection include warmth, redness, and swelling around the site; purulent or foul-smelling drainage; or a fever.
- In a systemic infection, a virus or bacteria has gained access to the bloodstream, spreading to other parts of the body as a result. Signs of a systemic infection include fever, malaise, nausea, vomiting, chills, and generalized weakness.

Bacterial and viral infection

- A bacterial infection is caused when bacteria are introduced into the body. The bacteria multiply to infect the patient, resulting in infection. Bacterial infection is typically localized. For example, a throat infection may result in worse pain on one side of the throat. Antibiotics can be prescribed to help kill bacterial growth.
- Viral infections occur when a virus invades through the mucous membranes. It attaches itself to a living cell and uses its genetic material to produce more of the virus. This results in the death of the host cell. Viral infections do not respond to antibiotic treatment. Though some antiviral medications exist, the usual course of treatment in a viral infection is to treat the symptoms and bolster the immune system to fight the infection.

Microorganism transmission
Microorganisms must move from one host to another in order to survive.

- Some microorganisms are transmitted via droplets that are released when an infected host coughs or sneezes. The microorganisms in the droplets can then invade a new host via the mucous membranes of the eyes, nose, or mouth. Microorganisms may also be transmitted through direct oral contact, such as through kissing an infected person or by drinking from the same cup as the sick individual.

- Iatrogenic transmission occurs when microorganisms move to a new host during a medical procedure, such as a surgery or line placement. On rare occasions, microorganisms can be transmitted through the fecal-oral route. This most typically occurs as a result of indirect contact with fecal material, such as through poor hand washing or by eating foods that have been contaminated.

Safety/Emergency

Preventing patient falls

Patient falls are a considerable problem in the health care setting. Injuries resulting from a fall are considered to be a primary cause of morbidity in older adults. The loss of coordination and bone density as people age puts them at an increased risk for breaking bones after a fall; the resultant loss of independence may lead to a decline in health and eventual death. Yet falling is not a normal part of aging. Proper prevention can greatly decrease a patient's risk of falling. As a nurse aide, it is important to follow fall precautions to prevent patient falls within the hospital setting.

Precautions to prevent falls
There are a number of precautions that can be taken to prevent patient falls.

- The first step of prevention is identifying the needs of the patient.

- If the patient has been determined to be a fall risk, a sign should be placed on the door so the staff knows the patient has special mobility needs.
- While the patient is in bed, at least two side rails should be kept in the raised position to prevent the patient from falling out of bed.
- Prior to standing with assistance, patients should be allowed to sit or dangle at the side of the bed to prevent dizziness that may result from the change in position.
- The patient should also wear rubber-soled shoes or socks.
- The floor should be kept free of all hazards, including puddles of water and small rugs that can cause slipping.
- While the patient sits in or stands up from the chair or wheelchair, the brakes should be kept locked.

Precautions for a bed-bound patient
Patients who are bedridden have a particularly high risk of falling.

- While the patient is in bed, make sure the side rails are up to prevent the patient from climbing out of bed.
- If necessary, a bed alarm may be placed in the bed to alert the nurse aide that the patient is attempting to get out of bed without assistance.
- The patient's call light should be placed within reach, as well as the patient's tray table and any other items the patient might need.
- Toileting should be offered at least every two hours, and the patient should be turned every two hours to prevent bedsores.

<u>Transferring the patient to the side of the bed</u>

Patient strength should be assessed prior to moving the patient to determine how much assistance may be required.

- While the patient is in bed, make sure the brakes are locked and the bed is in the lowest position. Lower the side rail, and raise the head of the bed until it is at a comfortable level for the patient.
- While facing the patient, place one arm behind the shoulders and one arm beneath the knees. Assist the patient into a sitting position at the side of the bed. Allow the patient to remain there for a few moments to ensure the patient is not dizzy from the change in position.

Transferring patient from a bed to a wheelchair: Care must be taken while transferring a patient from the bed to the wheelchair to prevent falling during the transfer.

- Prior to moving the patient, make sure the bed and wheelchair wheels are locked to prevent movement during ambulation.
- Ensure the patient is wearing rubber-soled socks or shoes to prevent slipping.
- Make sure the patient is not suffering from any dizziness or lightheadedness that may result from a quick change in position.
- Prior to beginning the transfer, explain the procedure to the patient.

Procedure for transferring patient from a bed to a wheelchair: move the wheelchair as close to the bed as possible, and make sure the wheels are locked. Lift the leg pads and footplates up and out of the way to prevent tripping.

- Explain the procedure to the patient.

- Assist the patient into a dangling position.
- Place your feet in a wide stance.
- Instruct the patient to stand on the count of three, and support the torso while helping the patient into a standing position.
- Pivot the patient so that his back is to the wheelchair.
- Instruct the patient to position his arms on the armrests of the wheelchair and back up until he feels the seat against the backs of his legs.
- Slowly lower the patient into a sitting position.
- Assist the patient in lifting his legs and placing the leg pads and footplates beneath them.

Transferring the patient from bed to a stretcher: While the patient is lying in bed, make sure the wheels of the bed and the stretcher are locked.

- Raise the level of the bed until it is the same height as the stretcher.
- If available, a slider board can be placed beneath the patient to facilitate movement and decrease friction.
- Stand at the side of the stretcher, and ask a colleague to stand next to the bed. Instruct the patient to cross his arms over his chest to prevent dragging his limbs across the bed.
- Grasp the draw sheet, and roll it to maintain a good grip.
- On the count of three, pull the draw sheet toward you, while the colleague at the side of the bed pushes the patient from the other side.
- Continue to pull until the patient is in the center of the stretcher.
- Position the patient for comfort.

Types of assistance

Stand by Assistance (SBA), Contact Guard Assistance (CGA), Minimum (MIN), and Maximum (MAX) assistance refer to the level of assistance the patient requires while ambulating.

- A patient who can move independently requires SBA. This patient does not require any assistance in ambulating and does not require a gait belt.
- CGA refers to a patient who does not require assistance but is at risk for falling. The nursing assistant should be close enough to touch the patient in case he should fall, but does not provide additional support.
- MIN assistance refers to the patient who needs a small amount of support while ambulating. A gait belt is advised for this type of patient.
- Patients who require MAX assistance may or may not be able to bear their own weight. This type of patient requires support from one or two staff members to ensure that he does not fall.

Technique for falling with a patient

Even with all necessary precautions properly observed while ambulating, the patient is still at risk for falling. A fall may result if the patient's legs give out from under him or if he were to lose consciousness while ambulating. If a sudden fall were to occur, it is important to protect the patient and yourself from harm.

- Support the patient using the gait belt and your free arm, and gently lower the patient to the floor or to a nearby chair, taking care to protect the patient's head.
- If the fall is uncontrolled as a result of loss of balance, focus on supporting the patient as much as possible while keeping you safe.
- Try to avoid tensing up prior to impact as this may cause additional injury.

Technique for ambulating a patient on crutches

The four-point technique is the preferred method of ambulation for a patient with poor lower body strength who is ambulating with crutches.

- While the patient is standing, instruct him to move the left crutch forward first, followed by the right foot. The right crutch should then be moved forward, followed by the left foot. The advantage of this method of ambulation is that the patient has at least three points of contact with the ground at all times, offering the most stability; the disadvantage is that it requires a slow movement speed.

The three-point technique is recommended for patients who are unable to bear weight on one foot while ambulating with crutches. While in a standing position, the patient should move both crutches and the affected limb forward. Then, while placing his weight on the crutches, the patient should move his strong leg forward until it is even with the affected extremity.

Swing-to method and the swing-through method of ambulation: The swing-to and swing-through methods of crutch walking are intended for patients who have decreased lower body strength. Both methods are advantageous in that they are easy to learn and allow for a quick gait. The disadvantage is that both methods require strong upper body strength.

- 17 -

- In the swing-to method, both crutches are moved forward and placed at the length of a step in front of them. The patient then places his weight upon the crutches and swings his body forward until his feet are equal to the crutches. In the swing-through method, both crutches are moved forward. Placing his weight upon the crutches, the patient swings his lower body forward and places his feet slightly in front of the crutches.

How a crutch should fit a patient: Though it is the job of the physical therapist to adjust crutches properly to the size of the patient, the crutch should be checked prior to each ambulation to make sure it continues to fit properly.
- The pads of the crutch should remain one to one-and-a-half inches below the axillary area.
- The handgrips should be even with the patient's hips.
- When the patient is in a standing position with hands resting on the handgrips, his elbows should be slightly flexed.
- When the patient walks on crutches, he should support his weight with his hands on the handgrips
- Placing his weight on the pads in the axillary area may cause nerve damage.
- The patient should keep the head and shoulders erect to limit back strain and keep the torso aligned with the crutches to prevent loss of balance and injury.

Transfer a patient from a chair or sitting position to a standing position using crutches: While the patient is sitting in the chair:

- Instruct him to hold both crutches in one hand by gripping the handgrips.
- Instruct the patient to scoot his hips to the edge of the chair and stretch the non-weight-bearing foot out straight.
- Help the patient rise to a standing position, using the arm of the chair to support one of the patient's arms and the crutches to support the other.
- Once the patient has balanced his weight on one foot, instruct the patient to move one of the crutches to the opposite side and place his hands on the handgrips.

Transfer a patient from a standing to a sitting position using crutches: To move from a standing to a sitting position:
- Instruct the patient to approach the chair until he is one step away from the front of the chair.
- Instruct the patient to carefully turn using his weight-bearing leg and the crutches until his back is to the chair.
- Assist the patient in finding his balance before transferring one of the crutches to the opposite side.
- Instruct the patient to grip both crutches by the handgrips.
- Help the patient to reach back with his free hand to find the arm of the chair.
- Instruct the patient to stretch the non-weight-bearing foot in front of him.
- Assist the patient with slowly lowering his weight into the chair.

Patient wearing a cast findings
Patients who are wearing a cast must be monitored closely to ensure they have continued circulation.
- If the fingers or toes of the extremity with the cast become cool, pale, or bluish in color, these

findings should be reported to the nurse immediately.

- Sudden severe pain, numbness, or tingling may be an indication of poor circulation or nerve damage and should also be reported.
- A foul smell or a burning sensation coming from beneath the cast may be an indication of infection, which should immediately be reported.

Technique for a patient with a cane

While ambulating a patient who is learning how to walk with a cane, always provide the patient with a gait belt.

- Instruct the patient to hold the cane in his strong hand.
- As the patient takes a step forward with the affected extremity, advance the cane forward, keeping the cane even with the leg and the patient's full weight upon his strong leg.
- Once the weakened leg and the cane are in place, instruct the patient to place his weight upon the cane while taking a step forward with the unaffected extremity.
- Allow the patient a moment to regain his balance before repeating the process.

Technique for a patient with a walker

A patient, who is learning to ambulate with a walker, should wear a gait belt at all times.

- Instruct the patient to stand in the middle of the walker, holding it by the handgrips.
- Instruct the patient to move the walker forward until the back legs are even with the toes.
- While keeping his weight on the strong leg, the patient should then take a step forward with the weaker leg, until it is in the center of the walker.

- Then, instruct the patient to place his weight upon the handgrips while taking a step forward with his strong leg.
- Once he has regained his balance, repeat the process.

Assisting a patient from a sitting position to standing with a walker: While the patient is sitting in the chair, open the walker and place it in front of him. Make sure the patient is wearing a gait belt.

- Instruct the patient to scoot forward until he is sitting on the edge of the chair.
- Instruct the patient to place both hands on the arms of the chair.
- On the count of three, assist the patient into a standing position.
- While providing support for the patient, instruct him to move his hands, one at a time, from the arms of the chair to the handgrips of the walker.
- Wait a moment to ensure the patient is not dizzy before beginning to ambulate.

Precautions to ensure safety during ambulation

While the patient is ambulating, make sure to provide support using a gait belt.

- Ensure the patient is wearing rubber-soled slippers.
- If the patient is receiving oxygen therapy, obtain a rolling tank so the patient can continue to wear oxygen while ambulating.
- Carefully monitor the patient's respirations, and frequently check to make sure the patient is not becoming fatigued or dizzy.
- Move at a pace that is comfortable for the patient, and do not try to rush him.
- If necessary, allow the patient to stop to take a brief rest in a chair to ensure that he does not become overexerted.

Precautions during oxygen administration

There are a number of precautions that should be taken to ensure the patient's safety while receiving oxygen therapy.

- The patient should be carefully monitored to ensure he is on an appropriate amount of oxygen.
- The patient and family members should be reminded of the facility's no smoking policy, as oxygen is highly flammable.
- Petroleum-based products should not be used while the patient is on oxygen, as these are also highly flammable.
- Care should be taken to make sure the patient does not become entangled in the oxygen tubing. Oxygen tanks should be stored in their appropriate holders; an oxygen tank can cause serious harm if it were to be knocked over and damaged.

Response when finding an unresponsive patient

Time is of the essence in treating a patient who is found unresponsive.

- If the patient is unarousable, call for help immediately.
- Check for breathing by leaning close to the patient's nose and mouth, listening for breath sounds, and watching for the rise and fall of the chest.
- If the patient is not breathing, administer two rescue breaths using an Ambu bag. Then check the patient's pulse.
- If the patient does not have a pulse, it is important to initiate CPR as quickly as possible.
- Lower the head of the bed, and place a backboard beneath the patient to ensure adequate compressions.

- Follow BLS protocols while attempting to revive the patient.

Response when finding a patient who is silently choking

Only initiate the Heimlich maneuver if the patient is conscious but unable to speak or make noise as this indicates that he is choking.

- Move behind the patient and wrap your arms around them.
- Make a fist with one hand and place it against the patient's abdomen with the thumb about 2 inches above the umbilicus.
- Wrap your other hand around your fist.
- Thrust your fist in and upward with as much force as possible.
- Continue to do this until the object has been dislodged from the airway or until the patient loses consciousness.

Ensure fire safety

Fire safety is very important in both the hospital and extended-care facility. Because of the presence of highly flammable materials, such as oxygen tanks, proper fire safety must be closely observed.

- The nurse aide should make note of the presence of oxygen shutoff valves, fire alarms, and fire extinguishers, and know the facility policy regarding fire alarms.
- Regular fire drills should be performed, and residents should be aware of necessary fire safety precautions.
- The fire extinguishers should be serviced regularly to ensure proper functioning.
- The nurse aide should also be aware of the facility code that indicates a fire. Though a fire is typically announced as a Code Red

on the overhead speakers, individual facilities may have different alarm codes.

<u>RACE</u>

RACE is an acronym that explains the proper procedure that should be performed upon discovery of a fire within the hospital or extended-care facility.

- The letter R stands for rescue. The first priority is to remove any patients who are in immediate danger from the fire. The nurse aide should only attempt to rescue a patient if she can do so without placing herself in imminent danger.
- The letter A stands for alert. Once any patients have been removed from danger, the nurse aide should activate the fire alarm system, if it has not already been done.
- The letter C stands for contain. Fire doors should be closed in an attempt to deprive the fire of oxygen.
- The letter E stands for extinguish. If it is safe to do so, attempt to extinguish the fire using the appropriate fire extinguisher.

<u>PASS</u>

PASS refers to the proper way to handle a fire extinguisher.

- The letter P stands for pull. A plastic ring keeps the fire extinguisher from being discharged accidentally. Pull the plastic ring off the fire extinguisher to ready it.
- The letter A stands for aim. Aim the nozzle of the fire extinguisher at the base of the fire.
- The first S stands for squeeze. Squeeze the trigger of the fire extinguisher to start the flow.
- The second S stands for sweep. Sweep the nozzle from side to side, covering the area of the fire completely. Continue to aim at the base of the fire, and do not stop the flow of fluid until the fire has been extinguished.

<u>Types of fire extinguishers</u>

There are three types of fire extinguishers that are typically found in a hospital or extended-care facility.

1. Type A fire extinguisher; it is typically silver in color and shoots pressurized water. Type A fire extinguishers are intended for ordinary combustibles, such as paper, wood, or cloth.
2. Type C fire extinguisher; shoots dry chemicals. It is typically red in color and is intended for fires started from an electrical source, such as a frayed wire or a piece of faulty equipment.
3. Type ABC or multipurpose fire extinguisher. These are also red in color and are intended for fires that have been started by either a combustible, liquid chemical, or electrical source.

Before using a fire extinguisher, it is important to make note of which type you are using; a Type A fire extinguisher should not be used on an electrical fire.

Emergency treatment for burns

Depending on the severity and the amount of body surface it covers, a burn can be a life-threatening injury. Shock induced by a burn and the resultant impairment of the immune system can cause serious harm to the patient.

- It is important to act quickly if the patient has been severely burned.
- A burn that extends over a small area of the body should be treated by running cool water over the affected area.
- A sterile dressing should be applied over the burn to protect the skin and to prevent the introduction of germs.

- Ice packs should also be applied to protect the skin and nerve endings.

Electrical safety

Proper electrical safety is an important step in fire prevention. The maintenance department should regularly service all patient care equipment.

- The nursing assistant should regularly check to make sure that all equipment is within its maintenance period.
- If a piece of equipment appears to be malfunctioning, it should be removed from service immediately.
- Prior to a piece of equipment of being used, it should be checked carefully to make sure its wires are intact.
- When plugging in a piece of equipment, make sure the circuits are not being overloaded.
- Also, closely monitor the floor near a piece of equipment to make sure there are no puddles nearby.

Good body mechanics

Proper body mechanics are described as the safe completion of tasks by using the appropriate muscle groups in order to avoid straining or injury. Health care workers have the highest incidences of work-related muscle injuries as a result of frequent heavy lifting, and these injuries are often slow to heal. Proper body mechanics are important in the medical field because of the frequent need to lift, turn, and reposition patients. Good body mechanics ensure the avoidance of using back muscles while caring for the patient, resulting in decreased fatigue and reduced risk of injury for both the patient and the nurse aide.

Principles of proper body mechanics
There are four principles of body mechanics that should be followed in order to avoid injury.

- The first is to maintain a proper center of gravity. This is done by bending and lifting with the legs and keeping your back straight as you are lifting.
- The second principle of body mechanics is to maintain a wide base of support, in order to maintain stability while lifting. Establish this wide base of support by keeping your feet at least 12 inches apart, with one foot slightly ahead of the other.
- The third principle is to maintain proper alignment. While lifting a heavy object, keep your back straight and the item that you are lifting close to you. If you need to turn with the object, pivot your whole body rather than twisting with the object.
- The fourth principle of body mechanics is to maintain proper posture while lifting. Keep your head up, your back straight, your knees flexed, and your buttocks tucked in to prevent injury while lifting.

Procedure for moving the patient up in the bed
Never try to move a patient up in bed by yourself. Always ask another nursing assistant or nurse to help you. Prior to moving the patient up in bed, explain to the patient what you are going to do.

- Wash your hands, and don a pair of gloves.
- Lay the head of the bed as flat as possible, and raise the level of the bed until it is a comfortable height for you.
- Position yourself near the head of the bed on one side, while the

other person moves to the opposite side of the bed.

- Instruct the patient to cross his arms over his chest to prevent his limbs from dragging and to tuck his chin to his chest. If the patient is unable to do so, support the back of his neck with one hand.
- Grasp the draw sheet and roll the edge to establish a good grip.
- On the count of three, lift the draw sheet and pull upward.
- Position the patient for comfort.

Applying restraints to a patient

Restraint policies vary from one facility to another, but their purpose remains the same.

- Restraints are applied in order to protect the patient from causing harm to himself or to other people.
- A restraint may be applied to prevent the patient from interfering with medical devices or moving in a way that would be detrimental to his health.
- It may also be applied if the patient is showing signs of aggression.
- A restraint should always be applied after all other alternatives have been exhausted.

It should not be applied as a form of punishment or for the convenience of the staff.

Different types of restraints: There are a number of different types of restraints that can be used in a health care setting.

- Emotional restraints are a method of using verbal or emotional cues in order to attempt to modify the patient's behaviors. This can include limit setting or contracting with the patient for safety.
- Environmental restraints are devices used to restrict patient

movement. These include side-rails on the bed or locked doors within the facility. When all four side-rails are in a raised position on the bed, it is considered to be a restraint.

- Physical restraints are devices that can be applied to the patient to restrict movement. These include wrist and vest restraints, lap belts, and movement pads.
- Chemical restraints are medications that are given to the patient to modify behavior.

Alternatives that must be pursued prior to the application of restraints: There are a number of measures that can be performed as an alternative to applying restraints. The type of alternatives that are utilized may vary depending upon the patient. Any needs should be assessed and all reasonable alternatives performed prior to application of restraints.

- The patient may need to be moved to a quiet environment.
- He may require more stimulation, such as hearing a television or radio in the background.
- He may require redirection.
- The patient may need toileting or water.
- He may need personal items placed within reach.
- He may require distraction if the care team is attempting to remove a medical device.
- If the patient has an illness or requires rest, it may cause him to act in a manner that is confused or inappropriate.

Prior to applying restraints to the patient: all other alternatives must be exhausted. The health care staff must attempt to identify and address the behaviors that require the application of restraints.

- An order from the patient's physician must be obtained in

- 23 -

order to apply restraints, and the physician should visibly assess the patient within 24 hours of the time of application of the restraints.

- Consent should be obtained from the patient's next of kin.
- Care must be taken to choose the least restrictive form of restraint.
- The type of restraint should be explained to the patient, as well as the reasons for the application of the restraint and the requirements for removal of the restraint.

Applying a vest restraint: A vest restraint is a device that is placed over the patient's chest to restrict movement. It is typically applied to prevent a patient from getting up without assistance. A doctor's order and consent from the family must be obtained prior to application of the restraint.

- The nurse aide should wash her hands and don a pair of gloves.
- She should greet the patient and explain the need for the restraint, as well as the requirements for removal.
- The vest restraint should be placed on the patient so that the opening is toward the back, with the straps crossing in the back.
- The straps should then be tied with a quick release knot directly to the chair or the frame of the bed.
- At least two fingers should be able to fit beneath the vest restraint to ensure that it is not too tight.
- Once the restraint has been applied, remove the gloves and wash your hands.
- Monitor the patient per facility policy.

Applying restraints to the extremities: Extremity restraints are applied to the arms and legs to restrict movement. A doctor's order and consent from the family must be obtained prior to application of these restraints.

- The nurse aide should wash her hands and don a pair of gloves.
- She should greet the patient and explain the need for the restraint, as well as the requirements for removal.
- The restraint should be applied per the manufacturer's instructions and tied to the frame of the bed using a quick release knot.
- The patient should be given a reasonable amount of slack in order to move.
- The nurse aide should be able to fit two fingers between the patient's extremity and the restraint; this ensures that is it not too tight.

Securing restraints to a wheelchair versus a bed: When securing restraints on a patient who is in a wheelchair, care should be taken to ensure the restraint is tied using a quick release knot attached directly to the frame of the wheelchair. The wheelchair should be locked, and care should be taken to ensure the restraints are not tied to the wheels.

- When the patient is in bed, the restraint should be tied using a quick release knot attached directly to the frame of the bed. Tying the restraint to the side rail can cause injury to the patient if the side rail should fall.

Proper procedure for monitoring a patient who is in restraints: Patients who are in restraints should be closely monitored to ensure safety.

- They should be checked every 30 minutes to make sure there is proper circulation.
- While they are restrained, patients should have their legs covered with a blanket in order to maintain privacy.
- The restraint should be removed every 2 hours to allow for range of motion.
- Patients should also be repositioned for comfort and offered water and toileting every two hours.
- Teaching regarding the restraints should be frequently reinforced to encourage patient understanding of the need for the restraint and the requirements for removal.

Therapeutic/Technical Procedures

Shaving a patient

Prior to beginning the procedure; wash your hands, greet the patient, and explain what you are going to do.
- Apply a pair of gloves, and use a wet washcloth to moisten the hair on the patient's face and neck.
- Check the razor to make sure it does not have any loose blades or jagged edges.
- Drape the patient with a towel, and apply shaving cream to the area that needs to be shaved.
- Use one hand to pull the skin taut, while moving the razor with firm strokes in the direction that the hair is growing.
- Rinse the razor in a basin of water as often as necessary.
- Use a moistened washcloth to rinse off all remaining shaving cream.

Performing hair care on a patient

Prior to beginning hair care on the patient, wash your hands, greet the patient, and explain what you are going to do.
- Don a pair of gloves.
- Raise the head of the bed to a comfortable level, and place a towel beneath the patient's head.
- Part the patient's hair into manageable sections, and run the comb or brush slowly through it.
- If the hair is tangled, hold the strand of hair above the tangle while combing it to prevent pulling the patient's hair. As you are combing, carefully inspect the scalp for any lesions, lice, or signs of dryness.
- Try to shape the hair into the patient's preferred style; even parting the hair on the correct side can provide a greater level of comfort for the patient.After hair care is complete, remove the towel and reposition the patient for comfort.

Nail care

- Prior to beginning nail care, wash your hands, greet the patient, and explain what you are going to do.
- Don a pair of gloves.
- Soak the patient's hands in warm water to soften them and prevent the nails from cracking.
- Carefully remove any dirt from beneath the patient's nails.
- Trim each nail by cutting straight across with a pair of nail clippers, then round the edges using an emery board.
- Be careful not to cut the nails too short as this may cause irritation to the nail bed.
- If desired, apply lotion to the patient's nails.

- After nail care has been completed, reposition the patient for comfort and wash your hands.

Oral care

Oral care performed on an unconscious patient as follows:

- Prior to beginning oral care on an unconscious patient, wash your hands, check the patient's name band, and explain what you are going to do.
- Don a pair of gloves, and drape a towel over the patient's chest.
- Adjust the level of the bed to a comfortable height, and raise the head of the bed greater than 30 degrees.
- Turn the patient's head toward you, and hold the mouth open with a tongue depressor in one hand.
- Clean the patient's teeth, gums, and tongue.
- After cleaning has been completed, suction the secretions out of the patient's mouth.
- Position the patient for comfort, remove the gloves, and wash your hands.

Oral care performed on a conscious patient as follows:
- Some patients may be unable to perform oral care on themselves as a result of palsy or weakness in the upper extremities.
- Before beginning oral care, wash your hands, greet the patient, and explain what you are going to do.
- Don a pair of gloves, and drape a towel over the patient.
- Raise the level of the bed to a comfortable height, and position the head of the bed greater than 30 degrees.

- Using a toothbrush, thoroughly clean the patient's teeth, gums, and tongue.
- While performing oral care, carefully inspect the patient's mouth for any lesions or signs of infection.
- If the patient is able to take small amounts of water without aspirating, allow him to rinse his mouth and spit the water into an emesis basin.
- Position the patient for comfort, and wash your hands.

Denture care is performed as follows:
- Prior to beginning denture care, wash your hands, greet the patient, and explain what you are going to do.
- Don a pair of gloves, and obtain the patient's dentures.
- Place a towel or washcloth in the sink to prevent breakage if the dentures are accidentally dropped.
- Using a toothbrush, clean the surface of the patient's dentures.
- Place them in a denture cup filled with cool water.
- Provide oral care to the patient using sponge swabs and mouthwash; carefully observe for any lesions or signs of infection.
- After the procedure has been completed, position the patient for comfort and wash your hands.

Bathing

Process for performing a bed bath as follows:
- Prior to beginning the bed bath, wash your hands, greet the patient, and explain what you are going to do.
- Fill a basin with water at a temperature between 105 and

115 degrees, and remove as much medical equipment as possible.
- Keep the patient covered to maintain dignity.
- Allow the patient to bathe as much of himself as possible.
- Begin by washing the patient's face, moving downward to the arms, the chest, abdomen, legs, back, and perineal area.
- Use a different washcloth for each area of the body.
- If necessary, change the patient's bed linens while washing the back.
- Apply lotion if desired.
- After the bath has been completed, reposition the patient for comfort and wash your hands.

Procedures for performing a tub bath as follows:
- Prior to beginning the tub bath, wash your hands, greet the patient, and explain what you are going to do.
- Make sure the bathtub has been cleaned.
- Place towels in the tub and on the floor outside the tub to prevent slipping.
- Ambulate the patient to the tub, observing all precautions.
- Once the patient is in the tub, fill it to the desired level.
- Make sure the water temperature is about 115 degrees.
- Provide privacy while the patient washes, but maintain close supervision to make sure the patient does not slip.
- Wash the patient's back and any area he is unable to reach.
- Drain the water, and dry the patient.
- Assist the patient into a standing position, and carefully help him out of the tub.

- Assist the patient in putting on his clothes.
- Position the patient for comfort, clean the tub, and wash your hands.

Procedure for perineal care as follows:
- Perineal care is an important part of bathing because it allows the nurse aide to inspect the skin of the perineal area. If done properly, it also decreases the risk for urinary tract infections.
- Perineal care should be done during a complete bath and should also be performed after the patient is incontinent.
- Wash your hands, and don a pair of gloves.
- Instruct the patient to open his legs.
- Cleanse the skin of the perineal area, using front to back movements.
- Never wash from back to front as this can introduce germs from the anus to the urethral area. After the skin has been cleansed, completely dry the area.
- Do not reuse the linens used to wash the peri area.
- Obtain a clean towel and washcloth to finish the bath.

Procedure for providing a back rub

Prior to giving a backrub:
- Wash your hands, greet the patient, and explain what you are going to do.
- Ensure that privacy is provided, and don a pair of gloves.
- If necessary, wash the patient's back with warm water and dry it completely.
- Warm the lotion in the basin of water, and apply a small amount to your hands. \

- Begin the backrub at the small of the patient's back, and work your way toward the shoulders using long, firm strokes.
- Use a circular motion when rubbing over bony areas to prevent irritating the skin.
- While performing the backrub, carefully observe the patient's skin for any signs of breakdown.
- After the back rub has been completed, position the patient for comfort and wash your hands.

Making an unoccupied bed

The linens on an unoccupied bed can be changed whenever the patient is out of bed.

- Wash your hands, and raise the level of the bed to a comfortable height.
- Lower all of the side rails.
- Place the fitted sheet on the bed, and pull it tight to make sure it does not wrinkle.
- Place the pad on the bed so that it will be positioned below the patient's hips and lower back.
- Carefully unfold the flat sheet, and place it on the bed, tucking the blanket so that the edges are mitered.
- Place the blanket on the bed, and fold the lower edge so that the corners are mitered.
- Fold the blanket and sheet back over the foot of the bed.
- Raise the side rails on one side of the bed, and put the bed back into the lowest position.
- Wash your hands.

Mitered corners
Mitered corners on a hospital bed prevent the sheet from being easily removed from the bottom of the bed.

- Place the sheet on the bed, and make sure there is an equal length of fabric hanging over each edge.
- Tuck the short end of the bottom edge below the mattress.
- Grasp one of the lower corners of the sheet and pull it taut.
- Pull it upward and at an angle toward the head of the bed so that it creates a triangle on top of the sheet.
- While keeping the corner taut, grasp the edge that is hanging over the side and tuck it beneath the mattress.
- Release the corner and allow it to fall into place, and then tuck the remaining fabric beneath the mattress.

Making an occupied bed
While the patient is turned on his side, undo the dirty fitted sheet and roll it toward the patient, placing the side that touched the patient inside the rolled up linen.

- Unfold the clean fitted sheet, and place it on the half of the bed that has been unmade.
- Place the pad on the bed so that it will be positioned beneath the patient's hips.
- Roll the clean linen, and tuck it beneath the rolled dirty linen.
- Turn the patient over the rolled up linen, onto the other side.
- Remove the dirty fitted sheet and pad, and place them in the soiled linen container.
- Unroll the clean fitted sheet and pad, pulling taut to ensure there are no wrinkles.
- Secure the fitted sheet to the bed. Roll the patient onto his back.
- Cover the patient with a sheet and blanket, and then miter the lower corners.
- Position the patient for comfort.

Indwelling catheter

An indwelling or Foley catheter is typically placed in patients who are unable to completely empty their bladder while voiding. It may also be placed for incontinent patients to protect their skin from the acidity of the urine. Post-surgical or critical care patients may receive an indwelling catheter in order to accurately measure their urinary output. The indwelling catheter is placed using sterile technique as follows:

- A rubber tube is threaded up the patient's urethra and into the bladder.
- A bulb at the end of the tube is inflated using sterile water; this keeps the tube in place and prevents leakage around the catheter.
- An indwelling catheter places the patient at an increased risk of developing a urinary tract infection.
- Catheter care should be performed frequently, and the catheter should be removed as soon as possible.

Caring for a patient with an indwelling catheter

Greet the patient, and explain what you are going to do.

- Wash your hands, and don a pair of gloves.
- Place the patient in a supine position, and lower the head of the bed.
- Place a water-resistant pad beneath the patient's hips.
- Using warm water, wash around the urethra in a downward circular motion.
- Never wash in an upward motion, as this may introduce germs from the rectum to the catheter.
- Wash around the indwelling catheter tube to remove any sediment that might be present.
- Carefully dry the patient's peri area.
- Hang the bag so that it is below the bladder, and make sure there are no kinks in the tubing.
- Never let the catheter bag touch the floor, as this can introduce germs into the bag and catheter tubing.
- Make sure the tubing is secured to the patient's inner thigh to prevent the tube from tugging.
- Once the procedure is done, remove the pad and cover the patient.
- Remove your gloves, and wash your hands.

Patient with an indwelling catheter: When a patient has an indwelling catheter, the urine should be checked frequently.

- The amount of urine drained from the catheter should be noted and reported to the patient's nurse.
- If the patient is not urinating enough (less than 30ccs per hour) or too much (greater than 400ccs per hour), the nurse should be notified.
- The appearance of the urine should also be monitored, and any abnormalities should be reported.
- Abnormal findings include cloudiness, sediment in the urine, or an unusual color, such as dark amber or green.
- The nurse should also be notified if the patient's urine is blood-tinged or foul smelling.

Placing a patient on the bedpan

Wash your hands, and greet the patient.

- Explain what you are going to do.

- Make sure the patient has privacy, and put on a pair of gloves.
- Lay the patient flat in a supine position, and turn him on his side.
- Place the bedpan over the buttocks, and carefully roll him back onto his back.
- Instruct the patient to open his legs, and make sure the bedpan has been placed properly.
- Raise the head of the bed, give the patient the call bell, and instruct the patient to call when finished.
- Remove your gloves, and wash your hands.

<u>Getting the patient off of the bedpan</u>
When the patient is ready to get off the bedpan:
- Ensure the patient has privacy.
- Wash your hands, and don a pair of gloves.
- Lay the head of the bed flat, and turn the patient on his side.
- While turning the patient, support the bedpan in order to prevent secretions from leaking into the bed.
- Remove the bedpan, and set it to one side.
- Provide perineal care for the patient.
- Position the patient for comfort, and allow him to wash his hands with a damp rag, if desired.
- Measure the output, and dispose of the secretions.

Tasks prior to providing the patient with a meal tray

Before taking the tray into the patient's room:
- Nursing assistant should check to make sure the patient is receiving the correct tray.
- Check the patient's armband and compare it to the name and room number on the tray.

- Check to make sure the patient's tray contains foods that are appropriate for the patient's ordered diet.
- Raise the patient's head of the bed, and place a towel over him to prevent bits of food from falling into bed.
- If the patient requires further assistance, cut any large pieces of food into bite-size pieces and open any containers.

<u>Procedure for feeding a patient</u>
Wash your hands, and raise the head of the patient's bed.
- Explain to the patient what foods are being served on the tray, and allow the patient to select what foods he will be fed first.
- When providing a bite to the patient, ensure the spoon is only half full.
- Use only the tip of the spoon to feed him.
- Feed the patient slowly, ensuring the patient has swallowed all of the food in his mouth before offering the next bite.
- Make sure the patient has had enough food to eat before taking the tray away.
- If the patient appears to be having difficulty swallowing, stop feeding the patient immediately and notify the nurse.

Tasks to be performed after assisting the patient with eating are as follows: After the patient has finished eating, remove the meal tray and calculate the amount of food the patient took in.
- If the patient is on a calorie count diet, calculate the percentage of food eaten and tolerance to the food.
- If the patient's intake and output is being monitored, calculate the

amount of fluid the patient took in.
- Report these findings to the nurse.
- Position the patient for comfort, and place the call light within reach.
- Make sure any necessary items, such as the tray table and personal items are within reach.
- Hand hygiene should then be performed.

Indications that the patient is not swallowing properly are as follows:
- A helpless patient is at a significant risk for aspirating food.
- During aspiration, small amounts of food and water move down the trachea and into the patient's lungs.
- Forceful coughing or a wet-sounding voice after swallowing a bite of food may be an indication of aspiration.
- If a patient needs to chew food for long periods of time or requires multiple attempts to swallow food, he may be aspirating.
- Other indications include unusual head movements while trying to swallow, difficulty breathing, drooling while eating, or pocketing food in the cheeks.

All of these signs should be reported to the patient's nurse.

Applying elastic bandages

Prior to applying an elastic bandage, check the order to confirm where the bandage is to be placed.
- Wash your hands, greet the patient, and explain what you are going to do. Apply a pair of gloves.
- Hold the end of the bandage in place with one hand, and wrap it around the extremity twice to secure it.

- Continue to wrap the bandage around the area that needs to be covered, working from bottom to top.
- While wrapping, overlap the bandages to keep them from sliding down and to ensure the area is covered.
- Once the elastic bandage is in place, secure it with tape, clips, or Velcro.
- Remove the gloves, and wash your hands.

Applying anti-embolism stockings
Prior to applying anti-embolism stockings:
- Wash your hands, greet the patient, and explain what you are going to do.
- Verify the anti-embolism stockings are the proper size for the patient based upon height and weight; they should be tight without cutting off circulation.
- Place the patient in a supine position.
- Gather the fabric of the anti-embolism stocking and slide it onto the patient's foot.
- Roll the stocking upward until the upper edge is placed above the patient's knee.
- Check to make sure there are no wrinkles in the stocking and that the stocking is placed properly so that the toes and heels are in the appropriate spots.
- Once the stocking is in place, position the patient for comfort, remove your gloves, and wash your hands.

Patients who are wearing elastic bandages or anti-embolism stockings: While patients are wearing anti-embolism stockings or elastic bandages, it is important to monitor them closely to ensure they receive an appropriate amount of circulation to their extremities.

- Frequently assess the patient's toes (or fingers, if the elastic bandage is on the arm) to check for signs of decreased circulation.
- Any complaints of numbness, tingling, or decreased sensation in the extremity should be reported to the nurse and investigated immediately.
- Make sure to remove the patient's anti-embolism stockings every 8 hours to allow for circulation.
- Elastic bandages should be removed per the doctor's order.

Range of motion on patients

Patients who are bed bound are at an increased risk of muscle deterioration from lack of use. Lack of regular exercise also places patients at risk for developing contractures, a painful condition that results in the permanent shortening of the muscle or tendon.

- Range-of-motion exercises can be performed to maintain muscle tone during periods in which the patient lacks the strength to perform other forms of activity.
- Patients may also be assisted with performing range-of-motion activities if they are unable to do so themselves, such as in cases in which patients are sedated or comatose.

Active range of motion and passive range of motion

Active range of motion (AROM) occurs when patients are able to perform range-of-motion activities by themselves. Though they may receive directions from the nurse aide, patients perform the bulk of the exercise.

Passive range of motion (PROM) consists of the same exercises that are performed during AROM. PROM occurs when the nurse aide is performing range-of-motion activities on a sedated or comatose patient to prevent muscle weakness. PROM may also be performed on patients whose muscle weakness is so pronounced that they require assistance in order to perform the activity.

Flexion

Flexion refers to bending at a joint, resulting in a decrease in the angle of the joint.

Extension

Extension refers to the straightening of a joint, or increasing the angle of that joint. For example, when the arm is bent at the elbow, it is flexed. When the arm is straightened, it is extended.

Abduction

Aduction refers to the movement away from the trunk. Adduction refers to a movement that brings a limb closer to the trunk. When the arm is moved away from the body, such as during jumping jacks, it is abducted. When it moves back toward the body, it is adducted.

Rotation

Rotation occurs when a part of the body pivots on a central axis. When the head turns from side to side, it is considered to be rotating.

Performing range of motion on a patient

Range-of-motion exercises are typically performed during the patient's bath. They can be performed while the patient is sitting in a chair or lying in bed. Each exercise should be performed 10 times to ensure it is effective.

- Wash your hands, and explain to the patient what you are going to do.
- Raise the level of the bed until it is a comfortable height for you.

- Begin by performing range-of-motion exercises on the patient's head; instruct the patient to rotate his head from one side to the other.
- This exercise should not be performed on patients who have suffered neck or spinal cord injuries.
- Work on the arms next.
- Flex and extend both arms at the elbow, then abduct and adduct the arm.
- Flex and extend both wrists and all fingers.
- Range of motion of the legs includes flexion and extension of the leg at the knee, as well as abduction and adduction of the leg.
- Finally, flex and extend the ankles and toes.

Abnormal findings to be reported if discovered while performing range-of-motion exercises: Range-of-motion exercises should be performed at least once or twice every day to make sure the patient's joints do not become contracted.
- Stiffness or the inability to move the joint may be an indication of the onset of contractures; if either of these symptoms is noticed, they should be reported to the nurse immediately.
- While performing range of motion, the nursing assistant should monitor for any signs of swelling or inflammation in the joints.
- If the patient experiences sudden severe pain or respiratory distress while performing range of motion, the nurse should be notified immediately.
  - Supine position: when the patient is in a supine position, he is lying flat on the back, with arms extended at the sides.
  - Prone position: a prone position consists of the patient resting on the stomach, with the head turned to one side on the pillow and arms extended at the side.
  - Sims position; when the patient is in the Sims' position, he should be positioned on his side, with both legs straight.
  - Lateral position: lateral position is similar to the Sims' position in that the patient is lying on the side. However, in the lateral position, the patient's topmost leg is flexed. Both the flexed leg and topmost arm are elevated on a pillow for additional support.
  - Semi –Fowler Position: the semi-Fowler's position consists of the patient lying on the back with the head of the bed at a 45-degree angle.
  - High Fowler : a high-Fowler's position is similar to the semi-Fowler's, however, the head of the bed is raised to a 90-degree angle.

Placing the patient in a side-lying position
Wash your hands, don a pair of gloves, and explain to the patient what you are going to do.
- Obtain assistance to help turn the patient.
- Raise the level of the bed to a comfortable height.
- Using the draw sheet, move the patient closer to the side of the bed opposite of the direction you

intend to turn him; this will allow the patient to remain in the center of the bed after having been turned.

- Grasp the draw sheet and use it to pull the patient onto his side.
- If the patient is able, ask him to grasp the side rail while you position him.
- Tuck a pillow beneath the patient's back, under the draw sheet.
- Tuck another pillow beneath the patient's buttocks.
- Place a pillow underneath the patient's arm and between the patient's knees for support.
- Remove your gloves, and wash your hands.

Logrolling procedure

Logrolling is a procedure that is performed whenever the patient has sustained a neck or spinal cord injury. Ideally, patients with this type of injury should be turned as little as possible until the neck or spine has been stabilized. In certain cases, turning cannot be avoided, such as if the patient has become incontinent. If the patient must be moved, the head, neck, and back must be kept in a stable position to prevent further injury. This requires good communication among the caregivers who are moving the patient to ensure that their movements are coordinated to maintain proper alignment. Logrolling a patient requires a minimum of three people in order to be performed successfully.

- Wash your hands, don a pair of gloves, and explain what you are going to do.
- Have one person positioned at the patient's head, and two others on the side in which the patient is to be facing.
- Grasp the draw sheet, and turn the patient.

- The person at the head of the bed should keep the patient's head midline with the rest of the body, while the people at the side of the bed keep the back and hips in alignment.
- Perform the necessary procedures, and then return the patient to his back.
- It is imperative that the patient's head, neck, and back are kept in alignment.
- Position the patient for comfort, and wash your hands.

Collecting a clean-catch urine specimen

Care must be taken while collecting a urine specimen to make sure that it does not become contaminated during the collection process.

- A clean-catch urine specimen can be collected from a patient who is able to void.
- Provide the patient with a sterile specimen cup.
- Instruct the patient to wash his hands and perineal area thoroughly prior to voiding.
- The patient should start the stream of urine and urinate for at least 2 seconds before beginning to collect urine in the cup.
- Don a pair of gloves.
- Once the patient has acquired a suitable specimen, close the specimen cup tightly and place it in a lab specimen bag.
- Encourage the patient to wash his hands.
- Remove the gloves, and wash your hands.

Collecting a urine specimen from a Foley catheter

When collecting a urine specimen from a catheter bag, care must be taken to ensure germs are not introduced into the

Foley tubing as this may cause a urinary tract infection.

- Wash your hands, don a pair of gloves, and explain to the patient what you are going to do.
- Clamp the catheter tubing 6 inches above the drainage bag, and allow urine to collect in the tubing.
- Thoroughly clean the collection hub with an alcohol swab.
- Carefully access the collection hub using a Luer-Lok syringe.
- Collect the desired amount of urine.
- Transfer the urine from the syringe into the specimen cup, taking care not to touch the cup with the syringe.
- Tightly close the lid of the specimen cup, and place it in a lab specimen bag.
- Unclamp the catheter tubing.
- Dispose of the syringe.
- Remove the gloves, and wash your hands.

Collecting a sputum specimen

A sputum specimen is often collected to check for infections in the patient's respiratory tract. To collect a sputum specimen:

- Wash your hands, put on a pair of gloves, and explain to the patient what you are going to do.
- Encourage the patient to cough forcefully to expel sputum from the upper respiratory tract.
- Instruct the patient to spit the sputum specimen into the cup.
- If the secretions are thin and clear, it may simply be saliva from the mouth; this is not an adequate specimen.
- Close the lid of the specimen cup tightly, and place it into a lab specimen bag.

- Remove the gloves, and wash your hands.

Collecting a stool specimen

A stool specimen is collected from the patient if there is suspicion of an infection or bleeding in the bowels. When the patient needs to move his bowels:

- Wash your hands, don a pair of gloves, and explain to the patient what you are going to do.
- Position a hat in the commode to catch stool without catching urine as well.
- Assist the patient to the bedside commode, provide privacy, and allow him to move his bowels.
- After assisting the patient back to bed, place a small amount of stool into a sterile specimen cup and close the lid tightly.
- Place the specimen cup into a lab collection bag.
- Dispose of the remaining stool and the hat.
- Remove your gloves, and wash your hands.

Procedure of putting on sterile gloves

Sterile gloves must be put on carefully to ensure germs are not introduced onto the sterile surface.

- Wash your hands, and dry them thoroughly.
- Unfold the package of gloves, and lay it on a flat surface.
- Using your nondominant hand, grasp the glove intended for your dominant hand at the fold of the cuff.
- Cup the fingers of your dominant hand, and carefully slide it into the glove.
- If the glove needs adjustments, wait until both gloves are on before making them.
- Using your dominant hand in the sterile glove, slide your fingers

beneath the cuff of the remaining glove.

- Carefully slide the fingers of your nondominant hand into the glove.
- Make any necessary adjustments.
- Do not touch any non-sterile surfaces, and keep your hands above your waist to maintain sterility.

Data Collection and Reporting

Five vital signs

The five vital signs that are most commonly measured are temperature, pulse, respiration rate, blood pressure, and pain level.

- Temperature measures the patient's core body temperature.
- Pulse measures the number of times the patient's heart beats per minute.
- Respiration rate measures the number of times the patient breathes every minute.
- Blood pressure is recorded as two numbers. The top number is referred to as the systolic pressure; it measures the pressure within the patient's arteries during contraction of the heart. The bottom number is the diastolic blood pressure; this number reflects the pressure within the arteries while the heart is at rest between each contraction.
- Pain level measures the presence or absence of pain. It indicates the severity of that pain according to the patient.

Oral temperature

Wash your hands, don a pair of gloves, and greet the patient.

- Explain what you are going to do, and check the patient's armband.
- Ensure that the patient has not had anything to drink in the past 15 minutes as this will make his temperature read falsely low.
- Cover the thermometer with a plastic sheath, and place it under the patient's tongue.
- Instruct the patient to keep his mouth closed and not to talk while the thermometer is obtaining a reading.
- Wait until the thermometer indicates the temperature has been read.
- Note the temperature, clean the thermometer, remove your gloves, and wash your hands.

How to take an axillary temperature
Wash your hands, don a pair of gloves, and greet the patient.

- Explain what you are going to do, and verify the patient's identity by checking his armband.
- Make sure that the area under the patient's arm is dry.
- Place a plastic sheath over the temperature probe.
- Position the thermometer in the axillary area, and instruct the patient to keep his arm down.
- Leave the thermometer in place until it indicates a reading.
- If a mercury thermometer is being used, allow the thermometer to remain in place for 10 minutes.
- Record the temperature, remove the gloves, wash your hands, and clean the thermometer prior to using it on another patient.

How to take a rectal temperature
Wash your hands, don a pair of gloves, greet the patient, and explain what you are going to do. Identify the patient using his armband.

- Place a plastic cover over the temperature probe.
- Assist the patient into a side lying position.
- Apply lubrication to the thermometer, and slide it 1 inch into the patient's rectum.
- Leave it in place until a temperature reads.
- If you are using a mercury thermometer, leave it in place for 3 minutes.
- Remove the thermometer, and inspect it to make sure it is still intact.
- Record the temperature.
- Position the patient for comfort.
- Clean the thermometer, remove the gloves, and wash your hands.

Indications of an abnormal temperature:
A person's core body temperature is closely regulated to ensure an optimum environment for the complex chemical reactions within the body. The normal temperature range for an adult patient is between 97.8 and 99.1 degrees Fahrenheit.

- A low core body temperature may indicate the onset of an infection. The patient's temperature may also be low after coming from a cold environment, such as the operating room.
- The primary cause for an elevated temperature is infection. Because a fever is the result of the immune system mounting a defense against an infection, it may not be necessary to treat the fever unless the temperature goes above 101.5 degrees Fahrenheit.

Apical pulse

An apical pulse measures the number of times the heart beats every minute by auscultating at the apex of the heart.

- Wash your hands, greet the patient, and explain what you are going to do.
- Verify the patient's identity using his armband.
- Place the bell of the stethoscope against the patient's left chest and locate the area in which the pulse is the loudest.
- If the patient's heart rate is regular, count the number of beats for 30 seconds and multiply by two. If the patient's heart rate is irregular, count the number of beats for a full minute.
- Record the patient's pulse, clean the stethoscope, and wash your hands.

Peripheral pulse

- Wash your hands, greet the patient, and explain what you are going to do.
- Check the patient's identity using his armband.
- Take the patient's hand, and slide your index and middle finger along the thumb, up to the hollow of the wrist.
- Apply gentle pressure until you can feel the pulse.
- If the patient's heart rate is regular, count the number of beats for 30 seconds and multiply that number by two.
- If the patient's heart rate is irregular, count the number of beats for a full minute.Record the number in the patient's chart.
- Wash your hands.

Indications of an abnormal pulse
The normal pulse range for an adult is between 60 and 80 beats per minute.

- The patient may have a low heart rate if he is physically fit or if he is resting.

- Some medications may also decrease the patient's heart rate.
- An elevated heart rate may be the result of exercise, stress, drugs, or caffeine.
- Certain medications may also elevate the patient's heart rate.
- If the patient has an elevated temperature or an infection, the heart rate will be elevated.
- An elevated heart rate can also be the result of uncontrolled bleeding.

Patient's respirations

Measuring respirations is done to assess the number of times per minute the patient breathes. Typically, when a person is made aware of his breathing, he does not breathe deeply or regularly.

- Do not tell the patient you are measuring the respiration rate, as it will make him aware of his breathing and may produce an inaccurate result.
- The ideal time to measure the patient's respiration rate is after checking the patient's pulse.
- Count the number of times the patient breathes, counting one rise and fall of the chest wall as one respiration.
- Count the number of breaths for one minute, noting the depth of the breath and any use of accessory muscles.
- Record the respiratory rate on the patient's chart.
- Wash your hands.

Indications of abnormal respirations
The normal range for respiration rate is between 12 to 18 breaths per minute. A number of factors may affect the rate of the patient's breathing.

- The patient may breathe more slowly if he is resting or if he is positioned on his back.

- Certain narcotics may also depress the respiratory drive, resulting in fewer breaths per minute.
- A rapid respiration rate may be caused by increased activity, pain, or stress.
- An elevated temperature or an infection may cause the patient's respiratory rate to be quicker.
- Other conditions, such as respiratory distress, fluid overload, or a heart attack, may also cause an elevated respiratory rate.

Checking the patient's blood pressure

- Wash your hands, greet the patient, and explain what you are going to do.
- Verify the patient's identity using his armband.
- Wrap the blood pressure cuff around the patient's upper arm, and place the bell of the stethoscope over the brachial artery.
- Pump the bulb of the blood pressure cuff, inflating the cuff between 150 and 180 mmHg.
- Slowly release the pressure, while listening through the stethoscope.
- Note the pressure at which you first hear a pulse; this is the systolic blood pressure.
- Continue to listen to the pulse.
- Note the pressure at which the pulse fades away; this is the patient's diastolic blood pressure.
- Record the findings on the patient's chart, and wash your hands.

Checking an orthostatic blood pressure
Orthostatic hypotension is a condition in which the patient's blood pressure drops as a result of a change in position. This can cause dizziness or lightheadedness

after standing, which may lead to falls. To check for orthostatic hypotension:

- Measure the patient's blood pressure while he is lying down.
- Assist the patient into a sitting position, and measure the blood pressure again.
- If the patient is able to stand, assist him into a standing position and measure the blood pressure a third time.
- If the patient's blood pressure drops by more than 20 mmHg systolic or 10 mmHg diastolic, then he is considered to have orthostatic hypotension. The nurse should be notified immediately.

Indications of an abnormal blood pressure

The normal range for a systolic blood pressure is 110 to 140. The normal range for a diastolic blood pressure is 60 to 90. Hypotension is defined as a systolic blood pressure less than 100 mmHg. The patient may have a low blood pressure because he is resting or as a result of certain medications. Bleeding, infection, heart failure, or dehydration may also result in hypotension.

- Hypertension is defined as a systolic blood pressure greater than 150 mmHg. The patient may have hypertension as a result of chronic illness, pain, or stress. Hypertension may also be caused by kidney failure, heart disease, or certain neurological disorders.

Intravenous therapy

An intravenous (IV) line is a small tube that pierces the patient's skin and rests in the vein. It serves as a method of providing the patient with medication and fluids.

- While receiving IV therapy, the patient should be closely monitored to make sure the IV line is in place.

- If the IV is leaking or oozing at the site, it may be an indication that the hub is not properly connected.
- If the patient complains of pain from the IV site coupled with warmth, redness, or swelling, it may be a sign that the IV line is no longer in the vein.

All of these signs should be reported to the nurse.

Measuring the patient's intake

In order to measure a patient's intake, the nurse aide must measure any liquids the patient takes in over a 24-hour period.

- This includes any water, milk, and juice the patient might drink, as well as any foods that melt at room temperature, such as ice cream, pudding, or jello.
- While measuring intake, the nurse aide should also include any tube feeding or any fluid that is used to flush a nasogastric tube.
- If the patient is receiving IV therapy, all IV fluids and medications suspended in IV fluid should be included in the patient's total intake.
- IV intake should also include any IV fluids that the patient received during surgery.
- Intake should be calculated in cubic centimeters (cc) and added up over a 24-hour period. That total should then be reported to the nurse.

Measuring patient's output

Output measures the amount of fluid the patient excretes during a 24-hour period.

- All urine should be measured prior to being discarded.
- The amount of liquid stool in a bedpan should be estimated prior to being discarded.
- If the patient has a nasogastric tube to wall suction, the nurse aide should note how much

drainage the patient has had out of the tube.

- If the patient has a wound that is hooked to suction, note how much blood has been removed from the wound.
- If the patient is having drainage out of a wound that is not to suction, the nurse aide should note how many times the dressing needs to be changed.
- Estimated blood loss from surgery should also be included as output.
- Add all secretions over a 24-hour period, and make a note of it on the patient's chart.

Observing the patient's bowel movements
After the patient moves his bowel:

- The nursing assistant should make careful note of the color and character of the stool.
- If the patient has multiple bouts of diarrhea, the nurse should be notified as this places the patient at risk of developing dehydration.
- Dark, tarry stools indicate the patient may be bleeding within the intestinal tract. Frank blood should also be reported.
- Furthermore, if the patient has not had a bowel movement in more than three days, the nurse should be notified as this places the patient at risk for developing constipation.

Intake and output calculation: After intake and output have been calculated over a 24-hour period, the two numbers should be compared. Ideally, intake should equal output as this indicates an equal fluid balance. Too much intake puts the patient at a risk for fluid overload, while too much output puts the patient at risk for dehydration.

- After comparing intake and output over a 24-hour period, the nurse aide should compare intake

and output over the past few days. This gives a better indication of the patient's ongoing fluid status. For example, a high intake on one day may be compensated on the following day with a high output, placing the patient's fluid balance at an equal level.

Measuring patient's height and weight

An upright scale can be used to measure the patient's height and weight if he has the strength to stand on the scale.

- Wash your hands, greet the patient, and explain what you are going to do.
- Confirm the patient's identity using his armband.
- Assist the patient to a standing position, and show him to the upright scale.
- Instruct the patient to stand on the scale, facing away from the scale.
- Lower the height rod until it rests on top of the patient's head.
- Make a note of the height.
- Assist the patient in turning until he is facing the scale.
- Move the weights on the scale until the bar is balanced; make a note of the patient's weight.
- Assist the patient back to the chair or bed, and position him for comfort.
- Wash your hands.

Height and weight measurement while the patient is lying in bed
A patient who is bed bound will need to have his height and weight measured while in bed.

- Wash your hands, greet the patient, and explain what you are going to do.
- Verify the patient's identity using his armband.

- Obtain assistance from a colleague.
- Roll the patient onto a bath blanket and the bed scale pad.
- Prior to obtaining the weight, mark the placement of the patient's heels and the top of his head on the bath blanket.
- Weigh the patient using the bed scale, and make a note of the patient's weight.
- Remove the bed scale pad and the bath blanket.
- Measure the distance between the two marks on the pad, and record that as the patient's height.
- Reposition the patient for comfort, and wash your hands.

Observations made while interacting with the patient

While interacting with a patient, the nurse aide must be vigilant to observe any changes in the patient's mental status.
- Check to see if the patient is alert or if he appears to be difficult to awaken.
- Assess the patient for any signs of confusion, such as disorientation to place or time.
- Make a note of any changes, such as increased weakness, slurring of speech, or the inability to follow commands.

If the patient shows any of these signs, the nurse should be notified immediately as these may indicate severe physical or neurological problems.

Data Collection and Reporting

If a change in the patient's status has occurred, the nurse aide should notify the patient's nurse immediately.
- The information should be reported in a succinct manner.

- The patient's name, as well as the room number and the bed number, should be included in the report.
- The nature of the problem should be explained, including the time of onset.
- The nurse aide should report any observations that accompany the problem. For example, if the patient developed confusion two hours ago, the nurse aide should include the manner in which the patient is confused.

Objective and subjective data
Objective data refers to information that can be referred to as fact. Objective data is quantifiable, such as vital signs, the patient's weight, or intake and output. Objective data also refers to anything that can be observed by another person. For example, if the patient has flushed cheeks, this is considered to be an objective fact.

Subjective data refers to anything the patient thinks or feels. The patient's pain level is subjective.

For example, the patient is developing a urinary tract infection. Objective data concerning that fact may be observations concerning cloudiness of the patient's urine. Meanwhile, patient's complaints of pain and difficulty urinating would be considered subjective data.

Purposes of charting
The purpose of charting is to create an accurate log regarding the care given to the patient, as well as the patient's response to the care.
- Items typically included in the chart are vital signs, intake and output, assessments, and procedure notes.
- Assessments are typically recorded on preprinted forms; any abnormalities in the patient's

assessment are included in the narrative notes. This is referred to as charting by exception.
- Notes are made in the patient's chart any time a procedure is performed on the patient.

Most information included should be objective in nature. Whether or not the nurse aide makes narrative notes in the chart is dependent upon hospital policy.

Principals of charting
While writing in the patient's chart:
- Write with only blue or black ink.
- Do not use a pencil.
- Write legibly, including only objective information.
- Avoid speculating or becoming overly emotional in the note.
- If an error is made, draw a single line through the erroneous information. Over the erroneous information, write "Error", the reason for the error, and your initials. Do not scratch out or scribble over the mistake. Do not use correction fluid to cover any errors.
- Do not edit another person's note or write over another person's writing.

Restorative Skills

Restorative care

Restorative care is given to an elderly patient to prepare him for meeting self-care needs after discharge. It is typically provided to patients who have been in the hospital for an extended period of time, such as after breaking a bone or emergent surgery. The type of activities provided during restorative care depends upon individual patient needs.
- Restorative care commonly focuses upon activities of daily living, including physical therapy, nutrition therapy, and occupational therapy.
- Emotional support is also provided to the patient to help treat the anxiety and depression that typically accompanies an extended hospital stay.

Home health care
Home health care is a service provided to patients who are healthy enough to go home but still require the services of a health care provider. The type of home health care provided is dependent upon the patient's needs.
- Services that may be provided to a patient by a visiting nurse aide may include assisting with daily hygiene, helping the patient to get dressed, cooking meals, feeding the patient, or range of motion.
- A nurse aide may provide other assistance, such as changing dressings, shopping for food, or taking vital signs.

Signs and symptoms of dehydration

Dehydration is a life-threatening condition that occurs when the body does not have enough water to perform normal body functions.
- Patients who are dehydrated may present with sunken eyes and dry mucous membranes.
- Dehydrated patients will often complain of generalized weakness and constant thirst.
- Their skin may lose its elasticity as a result of dehydration.
- They may have a weak, rapid pulse and a low blood pressure.
- The urine will become darker and more concentrated when patients are dehydrated; a result of the kidneys conserving as much water as possible.

Encouraging fluids on a patient

If a patient is dehydrated, he must increase the amount of fluids that he consumes in order to restore fluid balance.

- Explain to the patient why it is important to consume more fluids, and make sure a water pitcher and glass is within reach.
- Fluids should be encouraged each time you go into the patient's room.
- Also, make other fluids available, such as fruit juice or decaffeinated tea or coffee.
- Try to avoid sugary sodas or caffeinated beverages as these may not quench the patient's thirst.
- If the patient has family present, ask them to also encourage the patient to drink more.

Dehydration

Dehydration can be caused by too little intake or too much output.

- Limited intake may result if the patient is unable to take in fluid as a result of chronic nausea or difficulty swallowing.
- The patient may be unable to obtain an adequate amount of fluid if he is confused or kept NPO.
- Dehydration may also result if the patient is excreting too much fluid. The most common cause of over-excretion of fluid is frequent diarrhea.
- Excessive sweating from fever or exercise may also result in excessive fluid loss.
- Blood loss after surgery or a hemorrhage or fluid loss after a burn may also cause dehydration.

Signs and symptoms of fluid overload

If a patient is suspected to be in fluid overload, he should be monitored closely.

- The most significant sign of fluid overload is increased respiratory distress or crackles in the bases of the lungs.
- The patient may experience edema in the extremities, puffiness around the eyes, or fluid accumulation (ascites) in the abdomen.
- As the fluid accumulates, the patient may have an unexplained weight gain over a short period of time. A patient in fluid overload may have a bounding pulse, hypertension, or bulging veins.

If any of these signs are noticed, the nurse should be notified immediately.

Causes of fluid overload: Fluid overload can be caused by excessive fluid intake or by previous medical conditions.

- Excessive fluid intake can occur if the patient is receiving too much IV fluid or is taking in too much oral intake.
- The patient's intake and output balance should be closely monitored to ensure the patient does not continue to take in too much fluid.
- Sodium intake should be monitored as well as too much salt may cause an increased fluid absorption by the kidneys, resulting in fluid overload.
- Certain medical conditions, such as heart attack or heart failure, place the patient at an increased risk of fluid overload as the heart may not be able to accommodate an increased amount of fluid.
- Patients with a history of kidney failure may not be able to effectively compensate for fluid overload and should be closely monitored.

Constipation

Constipation occurs when the patient's stool is too dry and hard to be able to be passed easily, making him unable to have a bowel movement. The feces become dry and hard as a result of too much water being absorbed from the stool due to poor gastrointestinal motility. If the constipation is not treated, the patient may develop a bowel obstruction.

Diarrhea

Diarrhea refers to the frequent passage of loose or watery stools. Diarrhea places the patient at risk for developing dehydration because of the amount of fluid lost with the stool. Electrolytes are passed along with the fluid, which can lead to life-threatening electrolyte imbalances if not properly corrected.

Caring for a patient with diarrhea

Patients who experience multiple bouts of diarrhea are at a significant risk for developing dehydration.

- They should be closely monitored for any signs or symptoms of dehydration.
- The number of stools and amount of fluid that are passed should be monitored.
- A stool specimen should be collected as soon as possible to determine the cause of the diarrhea.
- If the patient is having frequent diarrhea, it is important to encourage him to drink fluids to prevent him from becoming dehydrated.
- If his diet allows, the patient should be encouraged to drink two glasses of fluid for every bout of diarrhea. Proper hand hygiene should also be encouraged.

Caring for a constipated patient

During hospitalization, there is a strong risk that the patient will develop constipation. This is often the result of decreased activity and the administration of medications that reduce gastrointestinal motility.

- The patient's bowel habits should be closely monitored.
- If the patient is using a bedpan, the consistency, color, and amount of stool should be noted after every bowel movement.
- If the patient is able to go to the bathroom without assistance, the nurse aide should inquire about the quality and frequency of the patient's stools.
- If the patient is constipated, it is important to encourage fluids to prevent drying of the stool.
- Warm liquids and juices are particularly effective in improving gastrointestinal motility.
- Caffeinated beverages should be avoided.
- Foods that are high in fiber should also be encouraged.

Urinary tract infection

The primary symptom of a urinary tract infection is painful or difficult urination.

- The patient may exhibit cloudy urine, which may have a strong or foul smell.
- The patient may experience the need to urinate frequently or may have sudden urgency in the need to urinate.
- The patient may also complain of flank pain or pressure in the pelvis.
- The patient may show signs of a generalized infection, such as an elevated temperature, flushed skin, or malaise.

- An elderly patient may also show signs of confusion as a result of the infection.

Prevention of a urinary tract infection
There are a number of ways that a urinary tract infection can be prevented.

- If a patient's diet tolerates it, oral fluids should be encouraged.
- Cranberry juice is particularly helpful in preventing urinary tract infections because it raises the acidity of the urine.
- If the patient needs assistance to void, help him to the bathroom as soon as possible as holding in urine can increase the patient's risk for developing an infection.
- While performing perineal care, the nurse aide should make sure to wash female patients from front to back.
- If the patient is able to ambulate, showers should be encouraged rather than baths.

Air mattress and an egg crate mattress

Pressure ulcers typically develop when the patient is unable to move as a result of illness or injury. As the patient lies in bed, his weight causes breakdown over bony prominences, such as over the shoulder blades and coccyx.

- When inflated, an air mattress decreases the amount of pressure placed upon the bony prominences.
- An egg crate mattress is a foam cushion that has alternating raised areas and grooves that decrease the area of pressure on bony prominences.

Though these items do not replace turning the patient, they can aid in preventing pressure sores in high-risk patients.

Prevention of pressure sores
There are a number of methods available to prevent the formation of pressure sores.

- The primary method of prevention is frequent repositioning.
- The patient should be turned and repositioned at least every two hours to prevent skin breakdown.
- Pillows may be used to provide additional support.
- The patient's feet should be elevated to prevent breakdown on the ankles, and the head of the bed should be kept at less than a 30-degree angle to reduce pressure on the buttocks.
- The patient's skin should be assessed frequently.
- The patient's nutritional status should be closely monitored as well since patients who have poor nutrition are at an increased risk of developing a pressure sore.

How pressure sores are treated: Pressure sores are difficult to heal as a result of the patient's compromised health status.

- If a patient develops a pressure sore, it is important to ensure it does not get worse by frequently turning and repositioning the patient.
- The patient should be placed on a support surface, such as an air mattress.
- This helps to decrease the amount of pressure on bony prominences.
- The skin over the affected area should be kept clean and dry.
- Dressings can be applied to the pressure sore, though the type of dressing depends on the severity of the pressure ulcer.
- It is also important to ensure the patient maintains good nutrition to ensure healing.

Caring for a patient with contractures

There are a number of treatment options for a patient with contractures.

- When a patient first develops a contracture, the nurse and the physical therapist should be notified.
- Attempts should be made to mobilize the joint using range-of-motion techniques.
- Heat therapy may be used prior to initiating activity to ease pain and increase flexibility.
- In some cases, the affected joint may be placed in a splint, which will continuously stretch the joint.
- Care of the splint should be performed as ordered by the doctor.
- If the contracture does not respond to other treatments, the patient may be taken to surgery to manipulate the tendon.

Edema

Edema can develop in the patient's extremities as a result of fluid overload or inactivity.

- The nurse aide can prevent swelling by encouraging the patient to move.
- If the patient is unable to walk, range-of-motion exercises should be frequently performed.
- While in bed or in the chair, the patient's legs should be elevated on pillows to prevent swelling in the lower extremities.
- Massaging the patient's extremities using lotion can also prevent edema.
- If the patient has a history of heart or kidney failure, his fluid and sodium intake should be closely monitored as too much can result in increased edema.

DVT and causes

A DVT, or deep vein thrombosis, is a blood clot that develops in the larger veins in an extremity. DVTs most commonly form in the legs, though the risk of developing a DVT in the arms does increase if the patient has an intravenous line.

- DVTs are most commonly caused by immobilization, though other factors such as obesity, infection, tobacco use, and advanced age can increase the patient's risk for developing a clot.
- The most common signs of a DVT include swelling and redness of the affected extremity.
- The patient may also complain of pain in the affected extremity.

Anti-embolism stockings
Anti-embolism stockings or T.E.D. hose are tight elastic stockings that are applied to the patient's legs. They are typically prescribed for patients who have undergone surgery or have decreased activity. When a patient is unable to move, blood pools in the legs, which increases the risk of developing blood clots and edema.

- Anti-embolism stockings work by placing pressure on the legs, which encourages blood flow. With improved circulation in the lower extremities, the patient's risk for developing a blood clot or edema is decreased. Care should be taken to frequently monitor circulation in the patient's legs while the anti-embolism stockings are in place.

Sequential compression device
A sequential compression device (SCD) is a pair of cuffs that are placed on the patient's legs to prevent the formation of blood clots. While the SCDs are on, the

device applies pressure to different parts of the legs over time.

- The increased pressure encourages blood flow within the legs, preventing blood clots. Care should be taken while the SCDs are in place to ensure the tubing does not become kinked as this prevents the SCDs from working. The circulation in the patient's feet should also be monitored. Frequent skin care should be performed as the skin underneath the cuffs can become damp and hot.

<u>Self-care program</u>
The purpose of a self-care program is to teach the patient how to provide self care after a long hospitalization or a debilitating illness.

- The focus of a self-care program may vary depending on the patient's areas of weakness. For example, a patient who has had a stroke and has weakness on one side of the body must be taught how to perform self-care activities safely and effectively.
- Self-care programs may include physical therapy, occupational therapy, and nutritional therapy.
- The patient may also receive assistance with medication management, food preparation, and other activities necessary to live within the community.

Clock method of feeding a patient

The clock method is a way of describing the placement of food on a plate to a visually impaired patient who is able to feed himself.

- The patient should be instructed to picture the plate as a clock face, with positions of food located at corresponding numbers. For example, the meat can be at the 12 o'clock position, the vegetables at the 3 o'clock position, bread at the 6 o'clock position, and the fruit at the 9 o'clock position.
- The nurse aide should try to repeat this pattern at every meal so that the patient is familiar with the locations of each type of food.

Bowel and bladder program

A bowel and bladder program focuses on giving the patient as much control over his bladder and bowels as possible. The purpose is to prevent incontinence by educating the patient on his bowel and bladder habits.

- Initially, the nurse aide should note the patient's voiding pattern in order to plan the patient's routine properly.
- The nurse aide should assist the patient in making note of the amount of food and fluid he takes in and help the patient to the bathroom at regular intervals.
- By establishing and reinforcing a pattern, the patient is less likely to be incontinent.

Aspiration precautions

Aspiration precautions are steps that are taken when a patient has difficulty swallowing to prevent food and drink from going into the lungs.

- Prior to being fed, the patient should be positioned with the head of the bed at a 90-degree angle.
- The nursing assistant should check to make sure the patient's food and drink is thickened to the prescribed consistency.
- The patient should be fed slowly, with the nursing assistant offering small amounts of food on a spoon.

- The patient should be allowed an adequate amount of time to chew and swallow.
- After the meal has been completed, the patient should remain upright for at least a half-hour to prevent reflux.
- After a half-hour has passed, the patient can be repositioned for comfort.

If patient begins vomiting in bed

If the patient begins to vomit while lying in bed:

- The nursing assistant should act quickly to make sure the patient does not aspirate on the emesis.
- The patient should immediately be turned on his side.
- A basin should be provided to catch any emesis.
- If there is a suction catheter, use it to clean any vomit from the patient's mouth.
- After the patient is done vomiting, allow the patient to stay on his side until he has recovered.
- Rinse the patient's mouth and face with cool water, and change the linens if necessary.

Psychosocial Care Skills

Orienting a patient to the facility

There a number of methods that a nursing assistant can use to orient a patient to a new facility.

- If the patient is only there for a short stay, it may only be necessary to orient him to his room. This includes orienting the patient to the bed controls; call light, and any continuous equipment he may be using, such as telemetry equipment or pulse oximetry.
- The patient should also be given any necessary information regarding unit policies and visiting hours.
- If the patient is expected to stay for a long period of time, such as at an extended-care facility, he should also be given a brief tour of the unit. If the facility allows it, the patient may benefit from being introduced to other ambulatory patients.

Dementia

Dementia is a term used to describe any cognitive dysfunction that may occur as a result of long-term illness, such as Alzheimer's disease, depression, and cerebral vascular accident.

- Dementia encompasses any resulting difficulties in memory, language, or problem-solving abilities.
- The patient is usually considered to be demented after six months of cognitive dysfunction; cognitive dysfunction that has gone on less than six months is typically referred to as delirium.
- Dementia may be curable, depending upon the cause.
- If the patient starts showing any signs of confusion, it should be reported to the nurse immediately.

Alzheimer's disease

Alzheimer's disease is a degenerative disorder of the brain.

- It is the most common cause of dementia.
- It typically affects people 65 years of age and older, though early onset Alzheimer's disease can occur.
- The cause of Alzheimer's disease is unknown.
- Initial symptoms of Alzheimer's disease include loss of short-term memory or forgetfulness.
- As the disease progresses, the patient experiences increasing confusion and aggression, while losing long-term memory, language skills, and other cognitive functions.
- Death typically results from breakdown of bodily functions.
- Alzheimer's disease is incurable; management of the disease is the key to an extended life expectancy after diagnosis.

Parkinson's disease

Parkinson's disease is a disorder that results in degeneration of the nervous system.

- It causes a decline in speech and motor skills and may cause a decline in cognitive function.
- Typical signs of Parkinson's disease include tremulousness, a shuffling gait, difficulty turning, difficulty speaking or swallowing, and a mask-like face.

- Parkinson's disease may also result in short-term memory loss and dementia in advanced cases.
- In most cases, the cause of Parkinson's disease is unknown, though in some cases the cause may be genetic or a result of a history of head trauma.
- Treatment includes medication management, management of symptoms, and surgery.

Causes of irreversible dementia

Multi-infarct dementia is the second most common cause of irreversible cognitive dysfunction. It is caused by tissue damage that occurs when atherosclerotic plaque on the vessel wall breaks off and migrates to another part of the brain, where it creates a blockage. Because the brain tissue cannot get an adequate supply of blood flow, brain tissue in the area of the blockage dies from hypoxia. Though the blockages can be treated, cognitive function does not return after treatment.

Huntington's disease is the degeneration of certain types of brain cells. Dementia often develops in the late stages of this disease.

Conditions that cause reversible dementia

There are a number of diseases and disorders that result in the onset of dementia.

- The most common cause of dementia is infection of the brain, such as meningitis or encephalitis. Both the infection and the resulting dementia typically resolve after treatment with antibiotics.
- Disorders that cause undue pressure on the brain, such as head injuries, hydrocephalus, and brain tumors, can cause dementia. There are treatments available to treat the increased pressure, and

the dementia diminishes after the pressure has been relieved.

- Disorders that affect other body systems, such as liver disease, kidney disease, or pancreatic disease, can cause dementia by upsetting the delicate chemical balance within the body. In order to restore the patient's previous mental state, the chemical balance in the body must be restored.

Sundowner's syndrome

- Sundowner's syndrome is a condition in which patients become increasingly confused in the late afternoon or early evening.
- It is most commonly seen in patients with a history of Alzheimer's disease or dementia; however, it can occur in patients who do not have a history of dementia.
- Though a number of theories exist as to why Sundowner's syndrome occurs, the actual cause is unknown.
- Patients who are suffering from Sundowner's syndrome may experience worsening confusion, restlessness, or agitation.
- Some patients may experience hallucinations or wandering as part of Sundowner's syndrome.

Steps a nurse aide can take to alleviate the symptoms of Sundowner's syndrome:
There are a number of steps a nurse aide can take to decrease the severity of Sundowner's syndrome.

- In the morning, the nurse aide should open the curtains and blinds and allow the patient to see outside to reorient them to time of day.
- Encourage exercise during the day.

- Plan all strenuous activities for the morning so that there is an adequate amount of time to relax prior to bedtime.
- Do not allow the patient to sleep during the day as this will make it difficult to sleep during the night.
- Plan a few relaxing activities before bed, such as therapeutic massage or quiet reading time.
- These activities should be performed at the same time every night to establish a routine.
- When it is time to sleep, darken the room as much as possible to further reinforce time of day.

Visual impairment patient

A nurse aide should take special precautions when caring for a patient who has a visual impairment.
- Prior to interacting with the patient, the nurse aide should acquaint herself with the type of visual impairment the patient has.
- She should make sure to identify herself as soon as she enters the room and stand within the patient's visual field while interacting with him.
- While ambulating the patient, the nurse aide should allow the patient to move as freely as possible and provide clear verbal cues regarding potential obstacles.
- The furniture in the patient's room should not be moved to allow the patient to become familiar with the surroundings.

Hearing impaired patient

If the patient has difficulty hearing in one ear the nurse aide should talk while standing on the side that the patient can hear.

- The nurse aide should introduce herself and speak slowly and clearly.
- The nurse aide should face the patient while talking to give him the opportunity to read lips.
- While talking to the patient, the nurse aide should try to limit background noise and deepen the tone of her voice in order to make herself better heard.
- If the patient can see well, communication can be achieved using written messages rather than speaking.

Aphasia

Aphasia is defined as difficulty speaking that results from lesions on the brain. Aphasia is typically caused by cerebral vascular accident, brain injury, brain tumors, or by progressive diseases, such as Alzheimer's disease or Parkinson's disease. Aphasia can come in a number of different forms.
- The patient may be unable to speak or may speak using inappropriate words and phrases.
- The patient may become unable to name objects or call objects by the wrong names.
- Aphasia can also affect the patient's ability to comprehend language.
- With aphasia, the patient may become unable to read, write, or form complete sentences.

Caring for a patient with aphasia: Prior to interacting with the patient, the nurse aide should acquaint herself with the type of aphasia the patient has and communicate with the patient accordingly.
- The key to caring for a patient with aphasia is to avoid becoming frustrated.

- Do not rush the patient; allow him time to gather his thoughts and say what he is trying to say.
- Avoid attempting to speak for the patient.
- Try to use a picture or letter board to assist with communication.
- If possible, allow the patient to write messages in order to communicate.

Mental changes involved in aging

Cognitive impairment in the elderly typically becomes noticeable at around 60 years of age, though the rate of decline varies depending on the individual.

- As a person ages, he typically experiences a mild decline in the ability to retrieve words and name common objects.
- Memory also tends to decline as a person ages.
- The ability to encode new information declines, typically as a result of a decline in sensory abilities.
- Short-term memory may also decline, though significant changes in long-term memory are typically not seen until about 70 to 80 years of age.
- The rate of memory decline can be stemmed using memory exercises and problem-solving skills.

Caring for a patient who is agitated
When a patient becomes agitated, the key is to remain calm.

- Remind the patient who you are, and attempt to reorient the patient to the surroundings.
- Speak calmly and clearly; attempt to learn what it is that is causing the patient to become agitated.
- Treat the patient as you want him to behave.

- While talking to the patient, assume a non-threatening posture.
- If possible, enlist the aid of family members to calm the patient down.
- If all of these measures fail and the patient is behaving in a way that may cause harm to himself or to other people, restraints may be required.

Caring for a patient who is confused
Confusion that develops in the hospital or extended-care facility is typically a symptom of a physiological problem.

- If the nurse aide notices confusion in a patient who was previously oriented, the nurse should be notified immediately.
- The nurse aide should try to find out what the patient's normal orientation was prior to entering the hospital; this can be done by reviewing records and talking to family members.
- The nurse aide should be observant for any signs of the physiological problem that may be causing the confusion. For example, cloudy urine may indicate a urinary tract infection, which could result in confusion in the elderly.
- Until the cause of the confusion is determined, the nurse aide should provide a safe, non-threatening environment while attempting to reorient the patient to the surroundings.

Reality orientation
Reality orientation is a set of activities that are performed with a confused patient in an attempt to reorient him to his environment.

- The first step of reality orientation is to approach the patient in a friendly, non-threatening manner.

- 52 -

While interacting with the patient, the nurse aide should provide verbal reminders regarding time and place. The nurse aide should provide the patient with physical reminders of the surroundings, such as writing the date on a whiteboard within the patient's visual field or showing the patient where a clock can be located.

Depression and its signs and symptoms

Depression is a disorder in which the patient experiences a consistently low mood, coupled with feelings of worthlessness, sadness, or self-loathing.

- The patient may experience insomnia (inability to sleep) or hypersomnia (sleeping too much).
- The patient may also complain of digestive difficulties or frequent headaches.
- Severe cases of depression may result in increased forgetfulness or hallucinations.

Depression can be caused by a number of physical, psychological, or sociological factors.

- Physical characteristics, such as a small hippocampus of the brain, may lead to the onset of depression.
- Depression may also be brought on by life-altering illnesses, such as Parkinson's disease, heart attack, or stroke.
- Tragic life events and the inability to effectively cope with them may also lead to an onset of depression.

Hospice care

Hospice care is a series of services that are available to provide end-of-life care for patients with terminal illnesses.

- Hospice care is typically made available to patients with a life expectancy of six months or less.
- A patient can receive hospice care at home, in a hospital, or in an extended-care setting.
- The purpose of hospice care is to help the dying patient to pass with dignity, while controlling pain and other symptoms and making the patient comfortable.
- The patient is cared for medically, while receiving spiritual and psychological support.
- Similar emotional support is provided to family members of the patient.

Stages of grief

When a patient is informed that he is going to die, he typically undergoes five stages of grief. These stages can occur in any order prior to acceptance, and the amount of time spent in each stage is dependent upon the patient.

- The first stage is denial. The patient is unable or unwilling to accept that he is going to die and often claims that a mistake has been made.
- The next step is anger. The patient is unable to deny the illness and reacts with resentment and anger.
- The following step is bargaining. The patient attempts to make a deal with a higher power in order to prolong life.
- Depression is the next step as the patient realizes that bargaining will not work to undo the situation.
- The final stage is acceptance as the patient realizes the situation and begins to make end-of-life preparations.

Priorities in caring for a patient who is dying

If a patient is actively dying, there are a number of priorities that should be kept in mind while caring for the patient.

- The patient should be kept as free of pain as possible.
- If the patient complains of pain, notify the nurse immediately so that the patient can be medicated appropriately.
- The patient should also be kept as comfortable as possible.
- Allow him to eat and drink what he wishes.
- Listen to the patient's concerns, and give emotional support to both the patient and the family.
- Allow the family to remain at bedside.
- Keep in mind that, even if the patient appears to be comatose, the sense of hearing is the last sense to fade prior to death.

<u>Caring for a dying patient</u>
Patient care should be provided as often as needed for a patient who is dying.

- The patient should be kept clean; if the patient needs to be bathed while the family is in the room, the family should be asked to step out while patient care is being performed. The only exception is if the patient asks certain members to stay or if his culture requires him to be bathed by family members.
- Oral care should be provided every two hours and as needed. If excessive oral secretions build up, the patient's nurse should be notified so the mouth can be suctioned gently.
- The patient should be turned every two hours. Vital signs are typically not ordered on a patient who is dying.

Signs and symptoms of impending death
When death is imminent, the patient will experience a significant change in vital signs.

- The heart rate will become slow and irregular and will feel thready when palpated.
- The patient's respiratory rhythm will become shallower, with the breaths becoming infrequent.
- The breathing may take on a rattling quality that results from mucous in the respiratory tract; this is referred to as a death rattle.
- Blood pressure and temperature will decrease.
- As a result of the diminished vital signs, the patient will become unarousable.
- Death typically occurs within minutes after the blood pressure is lost.

Providing support to grieving family members: If the family is not present when the patient dies, the nurse aide should make an effort to make the body look presentable prior to the arrival of the family.

- The body should be placed in a supine position and covered with a blanket up to the chest. If necessary, a clean gown should be placed on the body.
- The family should be given as much time as they need to view the body.
- The nurse aide should make an effort to offer comfort to the family, listening to them and providing emotional support where needed. The nurse aide should offer the family anything they might need, such as tissues or water.

- While viewing the body, the family should be afforded privacy by closing the curtain and shutting the door.

Postmortem care

Postmortem care is the process of preparing a body to be taken to the morgue.

- The nurse aide should make sure to treat the body with the utmost respect.
- Ensure privacy by pulling the curtain, wash your hands, and don a pair of gloves.
- If the patient has dentures, place them in his mouth.
- Close the patient's eyes.
- Wash the body as if performing a complete bed bath before dressing the patient in a clean gown.
- Place a pad over the perineal area.
- Remove any tubes and lines, and place a dressing over the line insertion sites to prevent oozing.
- If the facility policy calls for it, shroud the body in a sheet.
- Place the body in a plastic body bag by tucking it underneath in a manner similar to changing an occupied bed.
- Close the bag, tie the zippers shut, and slide the body onto a morgue cart using the assistance of one other colleague.

Rigor mortis

Rigor mortis is the stiffening of muscles that occurs after death, making the limbs very difficult to move.

- It typically occurs within a few hours after death and can last up to 72 hours after the time of death.
- It results from the breaking down of muscle tissue, releasing chemicals within the muscle that cause it to stiffen.
- Rigor mortis is significant because the patient's body can get 'stuck' if left in a certain position after death. For this reason, it is important to place the patient in a supine position as soon as possible after death.
- Certain facility policies call for loosely binding the patient's hands during postmortem care to prevent the limbs from freezing in unusual positions.

Culture

Culture is defined as the behavior and belief systems of a particular group. A person's cultural outlook is shaped by ethnicity, gender, and age. It affects his outlook on all things, including health care.

- It can affect the types of foods the patient might eat while sick, his behaviors during illness, and his attitude about death and dying.
- The patient's cultural beliefs should be taken into account when planning care.
- If the patient's cultural beliefs are not taken into account, it may increase the patient's stress level, hindering the healing process.

Religion

Religion is the set of beliefs that the person has regarding the nature of the universe.

- The patient's religion may dictate the level of participation in his care, including what treatments he may accept.
- Religion can also aid in the patient's ability to cope during the recovery period following serious illness or injury.

- The patient's religious outlook should be taken into account when planning the patient's care.
- Failure to do so may result in the patient's refusal to participate in the care or withdrawal from the hospital setting altogether.

Ensuring a patient's special dietary needs

Upon admission to the hospital or long-term care facility:
- The nurse aide should make note of any cultural or religious requests that the patient may have regarding dietary needs.
- The facility dietary service should be notified as soon as possible to ensure the patient is provided with appropriate foods.
- Prior to taking the tray in to the room, the nurse aide should check to make sure the food on the tray meet the patient's dietary restrictions. If it does not, the dietary service should be notified regarding the problem, and a replacement meal should be obtained as soon as possible.

Patient asks to see a priest

During times of illness or injury, it is not uncommon for a patient to request to see a priest or a person of authority within his church. If a patient makes such a request:
- The nurse aide should notify the charge nurse immediately.
- The charge nurse will talk with the patient and find out if there is a specific person the patient wishes to see.
- Most hospitals and extended-care facilities have an on-call clergyperson who can be notified if the patient does not have a specific person to call.

Considerations while caring for a Christian patient

It is important for the nursing assistant to ask if the patient has any dietary restrictions. Though most Christians do not have dietary restrictions as a result of their faith, some may have self-imposed dietary restrictions.
- Some Catholic patients may wish to fast during Lent.
- During their stay, some Catholic or Orthodox Christian patients may choose to receive communion or give confession during their hospitalization.
- Some patients may request to receive Last Rites if they are critically ill or dying.
- It is important to notify the charge nurse immediately if the patient requests to see a priest during his stay.
- In many cases, the patient or family will know a priest they would want to call.

Considerations while caring for a Muslim patient

It is important to ask the patient if he has any specific dietary restrictions. Many strict practicing Muslims will eat only specially slaughtered fish, chicken, and beef. Most Muslims will not eat pork products.
- Try to avoid handing a Muslim patient anything with the left hand as that is the hand that is reserved for performing perineal care on oneself. Muslims place a strong emphasis on cleanliness. Many Muslims prefer to wash with soap and water after using the bedpan, rather than using toilet paper. They should also be provided with fresh water to wash with prior to their prayers.

- 56 -

- If possible, female patients should be cared for by female nursing assistants.

Considerations while caring for a Jewish patient

Orthodox Jews eat only kosher meat and typically avoid dishes in which milk and meat have been prepared together. Other types of foods that are forbidden include pork products, meat from birds of prey, and shellfish.

- Most Jewish patients prefer to wash their hands and say a brief prayer prior to eating; the nursing assistant should provide them with an opportunity to do so. Jewish men may prefer to remain bearded or may choose to shave using an electric razor rather than a razor blade.
- Jewish patients observe specific practices regarding death. The family will notify their Synagogue of the patient's impending death; if there is no family present, the health care staff should do so. After the death, three members of the family typically wash the body. Burial should take place within 24 hours after dying.

Considerations while caring for a Hindu patient

- It is important for the nursing assistant to inquire about any specific dietary needs. Most Hindus are vegetarian or vegan; even those that do eat meat may refuse to eat beef or pork.
- After using the bedpan, most Hindu patients prefer to wash their perineal area using clean water rather than using toilet paper. The nursing assistant should make it available if requested. Some Hindus may

prefer to wash in the shower rather than sitting in the bath. Members of the Hindu faith particularly value privacy; if possible, the patient should be cared for by a nursing assistant who is of the same gender.
- Some Hindu patients may prefer to die while lying on the ground to maintain closeness between the individual and Mother Earth. If necessary, a Hindu priest may be called in to perform holy rites for the patient.

Considerations while caring for a Buddhist patient

It is important for a nursing assistant to inquire about a Buddhist's dietary needs on admission as many Buddhist patients are vegetarians or vegans. Many Buddhists fast on specific days, including the days of the New Moon and Full Moon. On fasting days, a Buddhist will only eat at specific times. The nursing assistant should collaborate with the patient on these days to ensure he gets his meal tray at appropriate times.

- The type of rituals surrounding death and dying varies depending on the patient's traditions. The patient may request a Buddhist monk or nun to perform chants in order to assist in the patient's passing. If possible, the body should not be touched until 3 to 8 hours after death before preparing the body for death.

Considerations while caring for a Mormon patient

Many Mormons follow a set of dietary restrictions put forward in the Word of Wisdom. It teaches against the use of stimulants, such as coffee, tea, and other caffeinated beverages. Though most

Mormons are not strict vegetarians, they do tend to eat meat sparingly.

- Some Mormons may wear a special undergarment that should be treated with the utmost privacy. It can be removed for laundering and washing but is otherwise worn at all times.
- Though Mormons do not have specific rites or rituals regarding a dying patient, the nursing assistant should make sure to allow the family to spend as much time as possible with the patient in his final hours. If the patient wears the sacred undergarment, it should be put back on the body after postmortem care has been performed.

Maslow's hierarchy of needs

A need is something that a person requires in order to maintain physical or mental well-being. Abraham Maslow determined the different levels of need that a person requires and organized them on a pyramid diagram.

- The first categories of need are physiological. These are the things a person requires in order to maintain life, such as food, water, and shelter.
- The next level is composed of those needs that pertain to safety and security. These are things a person requires in order to feel safe and comfortable in his environment.
- The next level is composed of love and belonging needs, which meet the person's desire to be loved and accepted as a member of a group.
- Self-esteem needs make up the next level of the hierarchy. These are the things a person needs in order to feel good about himself. The final level of needs includes those required for self-actualization, those things needed for a person to reach his full position.

Role of the Nurse Aide

Therapeutic communication

Therapeutic communication is a method of communicating with patients that encourages them to open up and provide information. Because of the level of stress involved in hospitalization, the patient often needs to communicate but is unsure how to initiate conversation with the health care staff.

- Therapeutic communication combines a variety of verbal and nonverbal communication techniques in order to encourage the patient to speak openly. By making note of the patient's body language as well as his words, the nurse aide can interpret the patient's emotional state and communicate with the patient effectively.

Components of communication
There are five components that must be present in order for communication to take place.

- The first component is the sender. The sender is the original source of the message.
- The next component is the message itself or what the sender is trying to convey.
- Another component of communication is the channel or the means through which the message is being conveyed. This is typically done using either verbal or nonverbal communication.
- The fourth component is the receiver or the person who is receiving the message.
- The final component is feedback or the response to the original message. The role of the sender and the receiver may interchange during the course of a conversation.

Verbal communication

Verbal communication is one way in which people communicate. It encompasses what is said as well as the way it is said. When communicating with the patient, the nurse aide should take into account:

- The patient's language and word choice, as well as the tone of voice and the volume at which the words are spoken.
- When talking with a patient, it is important to think carefully about what you say before you say it as words can often be misunderstood.
- It is also important to ensure that your comments are appropriate to the setting and conversation.

Nonverbal communication

Nonverbal communication is the process of sending messages using methods other than speaking. It can convey emotions and attitudes and can aid in communicating effectively with the patient. A person can communicate nonverbally using gestures, touch, or body language.

- A nurse aide should closely monitor her own body language to make sure that it does not contradict what she is saying. For example, a nurse aide who talks to the patient while frequently checking her watch is indicating that she is in a hurry. Such body language discourages open communication and should be avoided.

Encourage communication

There are a number of steps the nursing assistant can take in order to encourage communication with the patient.

- First, the nurse aide can ensure the patient is in an environment in which he can communicate freely. If the patient is comfortable, he is more likely to participate in therapeutic conversation.
- The nurse aide should also ensure the patient's privacy during the conversation. The patient may feel embarrassed about sharing personal information in a public setting.
- The nursing assistant should make an effort to appear unhurried, encouraging the patient to talk by sitting near the patient during the conversation.
- The nursing assistant should also convey interest by facing the patient and maintaining eye contact during the conversation.

Talking to a patient effectively

When the nursing assistant is talking to the patient, there are a number of ways she can make sure that what she is saying is clearly communicated.

- The nursing assistant should avoid using medical terminology while talking to the patient as many find it to be confusing.
- The nursing assistant should make an effort to use words that can be understood by the layman. For example, instead of saying 'hypertension', the nursing assistant can be better understood by using the phrase 'high blood pressure'.
- If a medical term must be used, the nursing assistant should define the term for the patient.
- While talking with the patient, the nursing assistant should speak slowly and clearly in a moderate tone of voice.

Silence as a communication tool

Silence can be an effective communication tool because it can convey a number of emotions. While communicating with the patient, silence can convey the sentiment of affection.

- This type of silence is typically accompanied by nonverbal actions, such as a hug or holding the patient's hand.
- Silence can also be utilized to encourage the patient to give more information. If this is done during a conversation, the patient may continue to talk to fill the silence.
- Silence can also give the patient time for contemplation.
- Care must be taken in utilizing silence as a communication tool as it can sometimes be misinterpreted as hostility or rudeness.

Active listening

Active listening is the method of listening attentively to the conversation at hand.

- During a typical conversation, it is not uncommon for a person to not devote her full attention to what is being said. She may be thinking of other things or focusing on the work she is trying to do.
- When a person is listening actively, she is not only paying attention to the conversation, but also considering the patient's words and forming an appropriate response that will encourage further conversation.
- Active listening also takes into account various aspects of nonverbal communication in order to draw the appropriate conclusions from the conversation.

Questions effective in encouraging communication

Asking questions can be effective in encouraging communication with the patient. There are two types of questions, open-ended and closed-ended.

- Open-ended questions encourage the patient to provide added detail about the subject of the conversation, while giving him more control over the conversation. "How do you feel about that?" is an example of an open-ended question.
- Closed-ended questions can be used to focus the conversation or get it back on track. They are typically used to elicit a short answer. An example of a closed-ended question is "What would you like for lunch?"

Encourage therapeutic communication

A general lead is a device used to encourage the patient to continue speaking about a particular subject. Examples of general leads include phrases such as 'go on' or 'I see.'

- These are effective because they allow the patient to guide the conversation, giving him the opportunity to voice his thoughts and concerns.
- General leads also indicate that the nurse aide is paying attention to what is being said.
- When a nursing assistant restates something, she rephrases a comment that the patient made earlier in the conversation in order to encourage the patient to elaborate on it. For example, the nursing assistant might say, "So you think you have too much equipment on you?" if the patient makes a comment about all of the tubes and wires attached to him.

Reflecting

Reflecting is another method of encouraging the patient to talk about a particular subject.

- A nursing assistant reflects a statement by repeating all or part of the patient's original statement back to the patient. For example, the patient says, "I feel so lonely." An appropriate reflective response would be "Lonely?"
- Another form of reflecting is to make a statement regarding the patient's feelings. For example, the nursing assistant may say, "It seems like you are very happy about this." This reflects the patient's emotional state and encourages him to speak openly about what he is thinking and feeling.

Providing information and self-disclosing

Providing information can be an effective tool in encouraging communication.

- When the patient is new to the health care facility, he may feel anxious about the unfamiliar surroundings. The nursing assistant can help ease anxiety by providing the patient with information that is relevant to his care. However, the nurse aide must be careful not to provide specific information regarding the patient's diagnosis or test and lab results.
- A nursing assistant can also encourage communication by providing some information about herself in order to ease the patient's discomfort. However, the nursing assistant must be careful not to dominate the conversation as the goal of therapeutic communication is to discover what the patient is thinking and feeling.

Touch and empathy

Empathy is the ability to understand what the patient is feeling and to respond appropriately. Acting empathically begins by recognizing any strong emotions the patient might be having. By recognizing these emotions:

- The nursing assistant can give the patient the opportunity to talk about his feelings, as well as provide validation.
- Acting empathically allows the nursing assistant to build trust and understanding with the patient.
- Using touch is a nonverbal method of communicating with the patient. There are times when words are not enough to provide an adequate amount of comfort.
- In these times, holding a hand or giving a hug can do more to encourage conversation and provide comfort.

Communication block

A communication block is a statement or behavior that discourages therapeutic communication.

- A nursing assistant may inadvertently use a communication block if she is hurried or is uncomfortable about the conversation at hand.
- Common communication blocks include the use of sarcasm or jokes in order to deflect the situation.
- The nursing assistant may change the subject or may attempt to minimize the problem in order to ease her own discomfort.
- Offering false assurances or telling the patient how he should feel in a given situation may discourage the patient from communicating with the nursing assistant.

Answering the call light

The call light is the way in which a patient notifies the health care staff that he is in need of assistance.

- It should be answered promptly and courteously.
- If a call light is going off in a room that is not assigned to you, it is appropriate to answer it to find out what the patient needs.
- If using an intercom, the nurse aide should answer by asking, "May I help you?" If answering the call light personally, the nurse aide should introduce herself and inquire about the patient's needs.
- It is not appropriate for the nursing assistant to ignore a call light if she is busy.

Patient continual use of call light

Frequent use of the call bell can occur for a number of reasons.

- The patient may not understand how to use the call bell or may push the wrong button accidentally.
- If this happens, a nurse aide can tape a piece of gauze over the button so that the patient can recognize the call button using his fingers.
- If using this method, it is important to check to make sure the call button can be pushed easily prior to leaving the room.
- Another reason that a patient may call frequently is that he is lonely. If this is the case, the nurse aide should make an effort to stop in to see the patient as frequently as possible. This may prevent frequent calls 'just to chat.'
- One way to prevent frequent use of the call bell is to make sure the patient has all necessary items within reach prior to leaving the room. Also, ask the patient if there

is anything else he might need prior to leaving the room.

If you do not know how to perform a procedure

Nursing assistants must perform a variety of tasks while caring for a patient. Some tasks may be performed on a daily basis, while other tasks may be rarely done.

- If a nursing assistant is assigned a task that she does not know how to do she should talk privately with the charge nurse after the assignment has been made to acquire instructions on how to perform the task.
- If there is still a question about how to perform the task, the nursing assistant should check the facility's policies and procedures manual.
- It typically contains an overview of how to perform a number of common procedures.

Patient's inappropriate comments

Some patients may attempt to use sexual innuendo jokingly or as a way to ease their own discomfort. However, such comments are considered to be harassment. Members of the health care staff have a right to work in an environment that is free of harassment. Some may try to diffuse the situation with a joke, but this approach is typically ineffective in halting the abusive behavior.

- If the patient begins making inappropriate comments, the nurse aide should immediately inform the patient that his comments are unacceptable and will not be tolerated. This should be stated firmly, but politely.
- If the patient continues the inappropriate behavior, the charge nurse should be notified.

Communication with non-English speaking patient

Patients who are unable to speak English may be a challenge to communicate with. Though it is possible to ask a family member to aide in translating, many facilities prefer to use an official interpreter when conveying medically related information to the patient.

- Whether communicating through a family member or an interpreter, the nursing assistant should look at the patient and address him while speaking.
- She should speak slowly and clearly, and watch the patient's body language and facial expressions closely as this can aide in the communication process.
- Before the family leaves, the nurse aide should ask them to write down a few common phrases, such as 'bathroom' and 'water,' to help with meeting the patient's needs.

Communicating with the patient's family

Interaction with the patient's family can occur frequently during the course of patient care.

- The nurse aide can confer with the patient's family regarding procedures that are part of the nursing assistant's scope of practice.
- When talking with the family while the patient is in the room, the nursing assistant should make an effort to include the patient in the conversation; it is inappropriate to talk about the patient as if he is not there.
- The nursing assistant cannot impart information about the patient's prognosis nor can she

give information about test or lab results.

- If a family member has a question about the patient's care, he should be referred to the charge nurse.

Unable to communicate with the patient

Sometimes the nursing assistant may be unable to communicate with the patient despite her best efforts. If the patient is intubated or has severe aphasia, he may not be able to effectively communicate his needs.

- The nursing assistant should attempt to figure out what the patient is trying to say by running through a list of common needs, such as being thirsty, hot, cold, or in pain.
- If the nursing assistant cannot figure out what the patient is trying to say, she should tell the patient that she is unable to understand him. She should not pretend to understand as this behavior can cause distress for the patient.
- The inability to communicate often results in frustration on the part of the patient. If this happens, the nursing assistant should provide appropriate reassurance and emotional support.

Patient's Bill of Rights

The Patient's Bill of Rights is a list of rights that the patient can expect to receive while he stays in a hospital or an extended-care facility. This list of rights may differ in wording from hospital to hospital but generally contains similar provisions.

- The Bill of Rights is typically accompanied by a list of responsibilities that the patient should adhere to in order to ensure his treatment is effective.

- It is important that the patient be made aware of his rights and responsibilities as soon after admission as possible.

The HIPAA act

Congress enacted the Health Insurance Portability and Accountability Act (HIPAA) in 1996 in order to ensure the privacy of patient health information.

- It requires each health care facility to prepare a list of policies and procedures in order to protect patient information.
- This includes limiting the ability to access patient information to only those who provide direct patient care.
- HIPAA also requires each health care facility to come up with technological safeguards to prevent the removal of patient information from hospital computer systems.
- If the hospital system violates the standards set forth by HIPAA, the hospital may be subject to severe fines and other penalties.

The right of privacy

Patients have a right to personal privacy.

- The nursing assistant should make an effort to protect the patient's privacy by maintaining his dignity during patient care procedures.
- While bathing the patient or taking him off of the bedpan, the curtain or door to the room should be closed to prevent other people from seeing in.
- The patient's right to privacy also applies to his health information.
- Details of the patient's case should only be discussed with the family members that the patient specifies.

- Many facilities have developed a system involving a privacy code number that is only given to the family members that are to receive information regarding the patient.
- Unless the family member is able to provide the privacy code number, the nursing assistant can only confirm the patient's presence on the unit.

The right of confidentiality

The patient has the right to have his case discussed only by those who are directly responsible for his care.

- Unless a nursing assistant is caring for the patient, she should not review his chart or discuss his case. Furthermore, once the nursing assistant is no longer providing care to the patient, she should not access his records.
- After the patient is transferred to another unit of the hospital, the nursing assistant should not access his files.
- Patient information should be discussed in areas where other people cannot overhear it to prevent laypeople from hearing details about the patient's care.

Right of respectful care

When a patient enters the hospital, he has the right to be treated respectfully by those who are providing care to him.

- The patient cannot be discriminated against because of age, gender, race, or religion.
- He also cannot be denied treatment as a result of the circumstances surrounding his hospitalization. For example, the patient cannot be denied care for injuries acquired during the commission of a crime.

- While the patient is in the hospital, he has the right to expect care to be provided safely by competent staff.
- While the patient is in the hospital or extended-care facility, reasonable measures should be taken to accommodate the patient's cultural or religious requests, provided they do not interfere with the care of other patients.

Right of informed consent

The idea of informed consent originally came about in reference to experimental treatment. However, it has come to encompass the type of information that should be provided prior to every test, procedure, or treatment.

- Before signing the consent form, the patient has the right to be informed about all of the risks and benefits involved in the proposed treatment, as well as the risks and benefits involved in refusing the treatment.
- He should be told which doctors will be involved in his care and what medications he will receive.
- The doctor should provide this information prior to the procedure, either directly to the patient or to the patient's health care power of attorney.

Right of freedom of choice

The patient's right to freedom of choice works in conjunction with the right of informed consent.

- Once he has been provided the necessary information, the patient has the right to choose what treatments he will receive.
- He is free to make this decision without pressure from the health care staff.

- Once he has made his decision, it cannot be undermined unless he makes the decision to change treatments.
- Conversely, if the patient decides to stop the treatment, he may do so, though the doctor should remind the patient about the risks and benefits involved in quitting the treatment.

Patient's telephone and mail rights

The patient has the right to have regular access to a telephone in order to communicate with family members.
- The patient should be informed as to where the telephone is located and how to use it.
- The patient should also have an expectation of privacy during his telephone conversations.
- The patient's conversations should not be monitored or recorded in any way.
- The patient has similar rights regarding the mail.
- Patient mail should not be opened without his consent, and any outgoing mail should be sent without being read by members of the health care staff.

Patient rights to see their chart

If the patient demands to see his chart, the nursing assistant should notify the charge nurse.
- Though it is the patient's right to see his chart, most facilities have a policy regarding patient chart review. Such a request is typically forwarded to the medical records department, who will make copies of the patient's chart to provide to the patient.
- This prevents the patient from potentially altering the information in his chart.

- Copies of the chart are typically provided within 10 days of the initial request.
- There may be forms for the patient to fill out prior to receiving copies of his chart, and the charge nurse or someone from the medical records department will provide the forms for him.

Do Not Resuscitate (DNR) order

A Do Not Resuscitate order outlines the type of heroic measures that may be undertaken if the patient's heart or breathing were to stop during the course of treatment.
- The DNR order typically specifies if the patient desires emergent intubation, CPR, or defibrillation. The doctor typically writes a DNR order after an extensive conversation with the patient about his wishes regarding his care.

In some cases, the patient may choose to have some of the emergency treatments, but not all of them.
- It is important for the nursing assistant to familiarize herself with the types of emergency treatment the patient wants.
- The patient can reverse a DNR at any time.
- If the patient verbalizes a desire to change his code status, the charge nurse should be notified.

Advanced directives

Advanced directives detail the patient's wishes regarding end-of-life care.
- They address whether the patient wants to receive long-term mechanical ventilation, continuous dialysis, or nourishment via a feeding tube.

- The advanced directives may also address whether the patient wants to be an organ or tissue donor after death.
- The patient typically sees a lawyer to have his advanced directives prepared prior to hospitalization.
- Health care providers should be made aware immediately upon hospitalization if the patient has advanced directives.
- If the patient's family brings in a copy of the patient's advanced directives, the nursing assistant should notify the nurse immediately.

Medical durable power of attorney

A medical durable power of attorney designates a specific person to make any medically related decisions if the patient should become unable to make the decisions himself.

- Durable power of attorney would take effect if the patient were to become confused or comatose.
- The durable power of attorney is typically filed by a lawyer prior to hospitalization.
- The person who has been made medical power of attorney should make an effort to learn the patient's wishes regarding health care decisions.
- If the patient becomes hospitalized, the family should present the durable power of attorney paperwork as soon as possible.
- If the patient's family brings in a copy of the patient's durable power of attorney, the nursing assistant should inform the nurse immediately.

Right to continuity of care

Continuity of care is defined as high-quality health care provided continuously and consistently. Often, continuity of care can be difficult to achieve in a health care setting because of the number of practitioners that can get involved in a patient's case. Continuity of care may break down for a number of reasons, including a doctor's lack of familiarity with a treatment plan or lack of communication among the health care team.

- In order to maintain continuity of care, there should be frequent conferences between the health care team and the patient to ensure that everyone is in agreement regarding the plan of care.

Patient's rights regarding experimental treatment

The patient has very specific rights when it comes to experimental treatment. Like any other procedure, informed consent is required prior to beginning treatment.

- The patient should be notified of the experimental nature of the treatment, as well as any potential risks and benefits involved in accepting the treatment.
- The patient should be approached in a manner that is not threatening.
- If the patient refuses the treatment, he has the right to be informed of other treatments that may be performed in place of the experimental treatment.
- Care cannot be refused to the patient based upon refusal of an experimental treatment.

Patient's right of refusal

If the patient is alert and oriented, he has the right to refuse any treatment or procedure.

- This includes simple procedures, such as turning or a bath.
- If the patient decides, for example, that he does not want to be turned, he should not be scolded or coerced for his decision. He should be informed of the risks involved in not being turned. If the patient continues to refuse, then the nursing assistant should not argue. The charge nurse should be notified so that the proper documentation can be made. If possible, the nursing assistant may offer the procedure again at a later time.

Patient insists upon leaving the health care facility

As long as the patient is alert and oriented, he may choose to leave the health care facility at any time.

- If the patient states a desire to leave, the nursing assistant should inform the charge nurse immediately.
- The charge nurse will talk to the patient and attempt to discover the reason that he wants to leave.
- If the patient cannot be convinced to stay and is considered competent to make that decision, the doctor will be notified of the patient's decision.
- In many cases, the patient will be asked to sign an AMA form, indicating that he acknowledges that he is leaving Against Medical Advice. It is not the responsibility of the nursing assistant to obtain the patient's signature.

Patient's right to the identification of health care workers

The patient has the right to know the names of the people that are providing care for him. On a given day, the patient may encounter a number of people, including doctors, nurses, physical therapists, and nursing assistants. A name badge clearly identifies a person as an employee of the health care facility and states the individual's position.

- It informs the patient of what to expect from the employee.
- When a nursing assistant enters the patient's room, she should wear her nametag above the waist in a location that is clearly visible. She should also identify herself in order to prevent confusion.

Patient's rights regarding money and valuables

Though it is unwise to bring a large sum of money or valuables to a hospital setting, it is sometimes unavoidable. Dentures and hearing aids, for example, are very costly pieces of equipment, but they are also necessary for everyday use.

- If the patient enters the hospital with money or valuables, he has the right to expect that the hospital will take reasonable steps to protect his property.
- The patient has the right to maintain his own accounts when he enters a long-term care facility.
- At no point should a member of the health care facility access the patient's financial accounts.
- If the patient is unable to take responsibility for his financial matters, the social worker should be contacted to make necessary arrangements.

Steps taken to protect patient valuables

If the patient comes into the hospital with large sums of money or jewelry, the patient should be encouraged to give it to a family member to take home.

- If a family member is not present, permission should be obtained from the patient to put the valuables in the hospital safe.
- If the patient consents, security should be called, the items catalogued, and a receipt given to the patient.
- If the patient is unconscious or comatose, the valuables should be locked up until he is able to give consent.
- If the patient has a valuable that is required for daily use, such as glasses, hearing aids, or dentures, every effort must be taken to protect these items.
- The patient should be provided a case marked with his name on it. When the items are not in use, they should be kept close at hand in a place where they are not at risk for breaking or being lost.

Rights of a dying patient

A patient's rights should be closely respected at all times, especially when he is dying.

- Every effort should be made to place the patient in a private room.
- When the family is present, the door to the room should be closed; if the door cannot be closed, then the curtain should be pulled shut.
- Reports regarding the patient should be given where others cannot overhear.
- Any monitor alarms should be turned off or silenced.

- Privacy should be respected if the patient needs to be cleaned up and during postmortem care.
- When transporting the body to the morgue, the morgue cart should be kept covered to protect the patient's identity.

Measures to protect the rights of patients with disabilities

Every effort should be taken to protect the rights of patients with disabilities.

- If the patient is hearing or visually impaired, the health care team should tailor its communication techniques to make sure the patient understands what is being said to him.
- If the patient is confused or mentally challenged, the patient's health care proxy must be kept informed of his status and conferred with regarding aspects of his care.
- If the patient does not have a health care proxy and there is no family available, a temporary proxy can be named to act in the patient's best interests until the patient is well enough to do so himself.
- If necessary, the health care facility's social work team should be notified to aid in protecting the rights of a patient with disabilities.

Patient's responsibilities

The health care facility must make every reasonable effort to provide treatment for the patient. However, an optimal level of health cannot be achieved without the assistance of the patient.

- The patient must actively participate in his care in order for treatment to be successful.
- Much like the patient's Bill of Rights, the list of Patient

Responsibilities should be provided to the patient on admission to the health care facility.

- These responsibilities include honesty and respect for health care providers, compliance with the treatment plan, meeting financial obligations, not putting others at risk, and responsible decision making.
- Failure to perform these responsibilities may result in the inability of the health care facility to provide adequate treatment.
- It is the patient's right to expect his health care providers to behave in a manner that is polite and respectful; the patient also has a responsibility to behave in a manner that is respectful toward his health care providers.
- Hospitalization is a stressful time for a patient; however, it does not excuse disrespectful behavior.
- Swearing, sexual harassment, and violence are unacceptable behaviors.
- Acting in such a way makes it difficult for the health care team to provide adequate care.
- If the patient exhibits behavior that is inappropriate, it should be addressed immediately to make sure it does not interfere with his care.
- It is also important for the patient to be honest when interacting with the health care staff.
- The patient should be forthright when answering questions regarding medical and social history as this information is vital in planning the patient's care.
- Without all of the necessary information, the planned treatment may be inadequate or may cause harm to the patient.

The key to maintaining a quality lifestyle is maintaining healthy habits. Healthy habits include a proper diet, exercise, and appropriate lifestyle choices. Though members of the health care team can provide information and encouragement regarding a healthy lifestyle, only the patient can make the necessary changes.

- It is the responsibility of the health care staff to review the treatment plan and provide education regarding necessary lifestyle changes. However, the treatment is only effective as long as the patient is compliant.
- If the patient chooses to refuse to follow the treatment plan, he must take responsibility if the plan were to fail.
- It is the patient's right to determine the type of care he receives.
- While it is the responsibility of the health care team to provide adequate information to allow the patient to make a decision regarding treatment, it is the patient's responsibility to make that decision responsibly.
- If there is an aspect of the treatment plan that is unclear, the patient should ask questions in order to seek clarification.
- It is also the patient's responsibility to make decisions regarding treatment based upon the information that has been provided to him, rather than basing his decision on emotions.

Standards of care

Standards of care provide a guideline that explains how a nursing assistant is expected to act in a given situation. The state government or the health care facility in which the nursing assistant is practicing typically sets these standards.

- It is the responsibility of the nursing assistant to be aware of the appropriate standards of care.
- If the nursing assistant were to fail to act appropriately in a given situation, she could be held responsible for any harm that might come to the patient as a result of her deviating from the expected way to practice.

Scope of practice

- Scope of practice is a list of tasks that a nursing assistant is allowed to perform as determined by the state certification board.
- It is the responsibility of the nursing assistant to be aware of what tasks she can and cannot perform. Any activity that does not appear on the list falls outside the nursing assistant's scope of practice; if the nursing assistant is caught performing an activity that is not on the list, she runs the risk of losing her certification.
- The nursing assistant is liable for any harm that comes to the patient as a result of the nursing assistant performing an activity that is outside her scope of practice.

Tasks not part of the nursing assistant's scope of practice
There are a number of tasks that fall outside the nursing assistant's scope of practice.
- A nursing assistant is not allowed to receive orders from a doctor; only a nurse can write orders.
- A nursing assistant may not insert or remove devices from a patient's body, such as indwelling catheters, IVs, or rectal tubes.
- Also, a nursing assistant may not perform any sort of sterile procedure.

- In most cases, a nursing assistant may not administer medications.
- Some states allow a nursing assistant to assist the patient in self-administration of medication under specific circumstances.
- The nursing assistant may only assist in medication administration if she receives special training and may only assist in administering certain medications.

Nursing assistant procedures when asked to perform out of her scope of practice
If a nursing assistant feels she is being asked to perform an assignment that is outside of her scope of practice, she should talk to the charge nurse privately after the assignments have been given.
- The nursing assistant should explain why she feels uncomfortable about the assignment.
- If necessary, the facility's policy and procedure manual can be consulted to confirm if the assigned task falls within the nursing assistant's scope of practice.
- If it does, and the nursing assistant still feels uncomfortable, she should request that the charge nurse be present while the task is being performed to ensure it is performed correctly.

Liability

Liability refers to the responsibility of a person to act within the confines of the law. In the eyes of the law, a person must take responsibility for his own actions.
- If a nursing assistant fails to perform a task to the best of her ability and harm comes to the patient, she can be considered liable.

- Similarly, if the nursing assistant performs a task that falls outside of her scope of practice and harm comes to the patient, she is considered liable.
- In order to maintain safe practice, it is important for a nursing assistant to perform tasks exactly as she learned them, without taking shortcuts.
- She should also make an effort to keep her skills and knowledge up to date with current health care trends.

Behaving in an ethical manner

Behaving in an ethical manner refers to doing what is right.
- In order to provide ethically appropriate care, the nursing assistant should strive to consistently provide high-quality care for her patients.
- In order for a nursing assistant to behave in an ethical manner, she must act in a manner that is in accordance with the standards of practice within her state.
- Behaving in an ethical manner also includes respecting the patient's rights, such as the right to privacy and confidentiality.
- Ethical behavior also includes remembering that not everyone behaves with the same values and ideals and respecting them for their differences.

Civil and criminal law

There are two different types of court cases: civil cases and criminal cases.
- Civil court cases take place between two people, when a wronged individual sues the person who did him wrong. If the accused is found guilty in a civil case, he is typically made to pay

fines and restoration to the wronged party.
- In a criminal court case, the defendant is accused of committing crimes against society as a whole. If a person is found guilty in a criminal case, he is made to pay fines or serve time in jail.

A tort

A tort is a wrong that is committed in a civil case. There are two types of torts: unintentional and intentional.
- In an unintentional tort, a person commits a wrong against another person without intending to cause harm. For example, if a nursing assistant forgets to put the side rails back up on the bed and the patient falls and injures himself as a result, that could be considered an unintentional tort.
- An intentional tort occurs when a person has the intention of causing harm to another person. An example of an intentional tort is if the nursing assistant leaves the unit without telling anybody, and the patient becomes injured while he is not being monitored.

Assault

Assault refers to the threat or attempt to touch or inflict physical harm on another person. The threat could be verbal or physical, such as a threatening gesture or advancing toward a person in a threatening way.
- Caution must be taken while caring for a patient; if the patient refuses a treatment and the nursing assistant attempts to force the patient to receive the treatment, she may be liable for assault. It is important to remember that the patient does

not have to be harmed in order for the nursing assistant to be found liable for assault. It is only necessary to prove that the patient felt threatened in a particular situation.

Battery

Battery refers to the act of touching a person without permission. It could refer to a violent act or an unintended act.

- A nursing assistant might also be accused of battery for performing a procedure on a patient without his consent.
- In order to protect herself from being accused of battery, a nursing assistant should take a moment to explain the procedure to the patient prior to beginning and obtain consent from the patient to perform the procedure.
- If the patient refuses the procedure, the nursing assistant should try to explain the reasons why the procedure is necessary but should not attempt to force the patient to have the procedure performed.

Negligence

Negligence is the failure to perform care in the manner in which that person was trained.

- A nursing assistant can be charged with negligence if she does not act in a way that is reasonable for a person with her level of training. For example, if the nursing assistant leaves a patient unattended in the shower and the patient falls and injures himself, the nursing assistant could be found negligent.
- A nursing assistant can avoid being accused of negligence by performing procedures exactly as

she learned how to do them, without taking shortcuts.

- If the nursing assistant is unsure how to perform a procedure, she should not hesitate to ask for assistance.

<u>Procedures for reporting negligent behavior of a co-worker</u>
The nursing assistant should be observant for any signs of negligence in the health care facility. Negligence can include failing to perform important tasks, such as turning or ambulating, or performing patient care activities in a manner that is unsafe.

- If the nursing assistant sees another member of the health care team behaving in a way that is negligent, she should report that behavior to the charge nurse.
- If it is the charge nurse who is behaving negligently, the nursing assistant should utilize the proper chain of command to make sure the behavior is addressed.
- She should not try to confront the negligent coworker herself.

Defamation

When a person makes statements about another person that causes damage to the individual's reputation, she can be accused of defamation.

- Slander refers to spoken defamation. For example, if a nursing assistant spreads rumors that a patient has HIV, that nursing assistant can be accused of slander.
- Libel refers to a written statement that causes injury to another person's reputation. For example, if the nursing assistant writes an article that a doctor is practicing without appropriate licensure and that article is untrue, she can be accused of libel.

A nursing assistant can avoid being accused of slander by avoiding saying negative things about other people. By spreading rumors, the nursing assistant is acting unprofessionally and places herself at risk for being accused of defamation.

Malpractice

Malpractice is a type of negligence that is committed by a professional who needs to maintain a license in order to practice. In a case of malpractice, a professional fails to act according to standards of care within her profession, which results in harm coming to the patient. Malpractice is more severe than negligence; it takes into account the professional's higher level of training when considering the wrong that was committed by the health care professional.

- Nursing assistants cannot be sued for malpractice as they are only required to maintain certification. However, they can still be sued for negligence.

Invasion of privacy

The patient has a right to keep details about him private. Invasion of privacy refers to failure to maintain the patient's right to privacy by relaying personal information without the patient's consent. The patient's privacy can be invaded if the nursing assistant shares details about the patient's health history with others or by inadvertently leaving sensitive documents where others can easily see them.

- A nursing assistant can avoid being accused of invasion of privacy by only discussing details of the case with those who are directly involved in the care of the patient.
- If a person who is not part of the patient's immediate family wants information regarding the

patient's treatment, the nursing assistant should refer him to the charge nurse.

Abandonment

Abandonment occurs when a nursing assistant leaves without notifying others or securing another person to provide care in her place.

- If harm befalls a patient while the nursing assistant is absent of her duties, she can be accused of abandonment.
- A nursing assistant can avoid being accused of abandonment by asking another nursing assistant to cover her patients and informing the charge nurse prior to leaving the unit.
- She should also make an effort to make sure all of her patients are safe and secure prior to giving report and leaving the unit.

Fraud

When a person commits fraud, she deliberately misrepresents herself for personal gain. It can be considered a violation of either civil or criminal law.

- A nursing assistant would commit fraud if she claimed to be a nurse or a doctor in the presence of a patient.
- It is also considered fraud to lie about one's qualifications or certifications on a resume in order to secure a job.
- A nursing assistant can avoid being accused of fraud by clearly identifying herself when dealing with a patient.
- She can also avoid being accused of fraud by acting within her scope of practice.

Theft

Theft is the removal of another person's money or belongings without his knowledge.

- A nursing assistant is guilty of theft if she takes a patient's belongings, even if the stolen item is not being used or is not of significant monetary value.
- Though the health care facility takes steps to avoid hiring people who might steal from patients, the nursing assistant should be vigilant as well.
- The nursing assistant should try to avoid theft by not leaving the patient's belongings in plain sight when they are not in use.
- If she sees someone stealing a patient's belongings or acting suspiciously, she should report the behavior to the charge nurse immediately.

False imprisonment

False imprisonment refers to confining a person to an area against his will. It is typically used in reference to use of restraints. Restraints are an acceptable tool to be used as a last resort in order to protect both the patient and the safety of others.

- False imprisonment refers to the use of restraints without an order or in a situation in which it is inappropriate to restrain the patient.
- A patient could also be falsely imprisoned if he is confined to the health care facility when he wishes to leave.
- If the patient expresses a desire to leave the hospital and he is alert and able to make decisions for himself, the nursing assistant should avoid attempting to force the patient to stay. Instead, she

should notify the charge nurse or the supervisor immediately.

Abuse

Abuse is any sort of action that results in the physical harm, mental harm, or death of the patient. It is a criminal act and most typically results in imprisonment. Abusive actions can be deliberate or can be the result of negligence. It can take a number of forms, including physical, psychological, verbal, sexual, or financial abuse. Abuse can be subtle, and some victims of abuse may be reluctant to come forward. The nursing assistant should be vigilant for any signs of abuse and report any findings to the charge nurse immediately.

Psychological abuse
Psychological or emotional abuse occurs when a person uses psychological attacks in order to intimidate or humiliate another person. It is typically done in order to coerce the person into doing something that he does not want to do. Psychological abuse can include teasing, threatening harm, or abandonment.

- Psychological abuse can be difficult to identify because it does not necessarily leave physical marks.
- Person who has been psychologically abused may show vague symptoms, such as chronic depression, anxiety, anger, or posttraumatic stress disorder.
- In many cases, other types of abuse accompany psychological abuse.

Verbal abuse
Verbal abuse refers to using words and threats in order to demean or upset another person. Verbal abuse includes threatening another person, raising one's voice in anger, or using profanity or

derogatory statements toward the other person.

- It can be difficult to identify a person who is being verbally abused.
- They may complain of vague symptoms, such as depression, anxiety, anger, or a feeling of hopelessness.
- In many cases, the victim may blame himself or herself for the abuse or may be overcome with hopelessness that the abuse cannot be stopped.
- Verbal abuse is often accompanied by physical abuse.

Financial abuse
Financial abuse occurs when a person takes the money and belongings of another person. The elderly are most commonly the victims of financial abuse. Forms of financial abuse include forcing a person to sign over property, using monthly disability checks for items other than the elderly person's care, or forging another person's signature.

- Being observant is the best way to catch financial abuse.
- It is possible that the patient is being abused financially if the patient lacks basic amenities, such as appropriate clothing or necessary personal items, (e.g. glasses or hearing aids) despite adequate financial assistance.

Physical abuse
Physical abuse is the most obvious form of abuse. It occurs when one person deliberately inflicts harm on another person and may be accompanied by verbal, emotional, or sexual abuse.

- Signs of physical abuse include bruising or abrasions with a distinctive shape, such as a fist or foot.
- Any injuries that do not coincide with the provided explanation

should be suspected. For example, a caregiver states that the patient burned himself while cooking.
- The explanation would be suspect if the burns are in a suspicious place, such as on the inner arm or on the abdomen.
- If a caregiver refuses to leave the patient's side during an interview or insists upon speaking for the patient, this behavior should also be suspected.

Sexual abuse
Sexual abuse is any unwanted sexual behavior directed from one person to another. It includes any sexually suggestive comments or gestures, unwanted touching or fondling, or coercion to perform a sexual act. Additional forms of sexual abuse include sexual harassment or behavior that is sexually demeaning. Other forms of abuse may accompany sexual abuse in order to frighten the victim into maintaining silence.

- Possible signs of sexual abuse include bruising around the perineal area, complaints of abdominal pain, or reoccurring yeast or urinary tract infections.
- The patient may also exhibit depression or increased anxiety or anger.

Procedures if a nursing assistant suspects that a member of the patient's family is abusing the patient.
It is the obligation of the health care facility to report any incidences of abuse to the state in order to protect the victim and remove him from the situation.

- The nursing assistant should be vigilant for any signs of abuse and should report any signs of abuse to the charge nurse.
- This includes any physical signs of abuse, any statements made by the patient regarding abuse, or

any signs of neglect. Once the findings have been reported to the charge nurse, the health care team will determine if any a
- buse has taken place and notify the proper authorities.
- The nursing assistant should not try to discuss the subject with the victim by herself, and she should not attempt to confront or accuse the abuser.

Nursing assistant procedures if she becomes frustrated: In many cases of abuse, the caregiver is responsible for inflicting the abuse on the patient. The abusive behavior may stem from feelings of exhaustion or frustration related to caring for another person.

- Nursing assistants can also feel this type of frustration.
- Whenever a nursing assistant finds herself becoming frustrated with a person or situation, she should remove herself from the situation as quickly as possible.
- She should take a moment to try and recognize the source of her frustration.
- She might find it helpful to talk to the charge nurse about her feelings or try to work with a different team of patients on her next shift.
- If these measures do not work, it would be beneficial for the nursing assistant to seek counseling through her job, to protect herself and her patients.

What a nursing assistant should do if a patient offers her a tip for her services: In some cases, the patient may attempt to give the nursing assistant a tip for her services by offering money or small gifts.

- The nursing assistant should politely and firmly refuse these offers.
- She should explain to the patient that he is being charged by the health care facility for all services that are provided, and the nursing assistant's pay is included in that fee. Usually, one refusal is enough to satisfy the patient.
- If the patient persists, the nursing assistant should remain firm and continue to politely refuse any offers of gifts.

Certified nursing assistant role

A nursing assistant is a valuable member of the health care team. Her primary role is to assist the nurse in providing care for the patient. The nursing assistant's primary responsibility is to see to the patient's basic needs.

- The requirements to become certified as a nursing assistant vary depending upon the state. However, most states require a minimum of 75 hours of training, including classroom instruction and review of basic skills. After the training has been completed, a nursing assistant must undergo the state certification exam in order to be qualified to provide care to patients. The test is typically divided into two parts, a written exam and a demonstration of skills.

Importance of continuing education

Unless a nursing assistant continues to study and learn, her skills will become outdated.

- The health care facility is required to provide at least 12 hours of continuing education every year in order for the nursing assistant to keep her skills up to date.
- Continuing education includes teaching regarding new skills and

a review of skills that are already known.

- It is the responsibility of the nursing assistant to provide proof of continuing education in order to maintain certification.
- If the facility does not offer it, the nursing assistant should speak to her supervisor about what she can do to acquire her continuing education hours.

Members of the health care team

The health care team is a group of people who provide care for a patient. It includes the patient, the physician, the nurse and other members of the nursing team, and any specialists who may be brought in to aid in caring for the patient.

- The patient is the most important member of the health care team; he consents to any treatments that might be performed and must actively participate in order for treatment to be successful.
- The physician diagnoses any diseases or conditions the patient may have and prescribes medications and treatments to treat the patient.
- The nurse is responsible for assessing the patient and administering medications.
- The nursing assistant aids the nurse in providing care to the patient.
- Specialists may be consulted to aid in the patient's treatment, such as a physical therapist or a speech therapist.

Set up of a patient's room

It is important for a patient's room to be properly set up prior to his arrival. This ensures the admission process goes as smoothly as possible. When the nursing assistant receives word of an admission,

she should make sure the room is set up as soon as possible.

- The bed linens should be turned down.
- There should be a clean hospital gown in the room in case the patient arrives wearing street clothes or a soiled gown.
- The room supplies should be stocked.
- Telemetry equipment and other necessary equipment should be at bedside; this can include a thermometer, sphygmomanometer, or pulse oximetry probe.
- Miscellaneous equipment, such as oxygen tubing, Foley catheter equipment, a graduated cylinder, and suction equipment should be provided if it is ordered.
- The nursing assistant should also have the packet of admission paperwork at the bedside.

Dressing for a job interview

A job interview is the first opportunity for a prospective employer to meet an interviewee. It is important to create a good first impression.

- The interviewee's clothes should be neat and pressed.
- Female interviewees should wear a skirt or slacks and a blouse.
- Any makeup should be carefully done so that it is not too heavy.
- Female applicants should also avoid wearing too much jewelry.
- Male applicants should wear a dress shirt and slacks.
- Shoes should be polished and not scuffed.
- Nails should be neatly trimmed, and hair should be well groomed.

Topics to discuss during a job interview
A job interview is a time for an interviewer to meet an applicant, but it is

also a good time for an applicant to get to know the interviewer and the place in which she will be working.

- Before the interview, the nursing assistant should think of questions regarding the job description and the facility and write them down.
- This might include questions about the nurse/patient ratio and the most common types of patients that receive care at the facility.
- It might also include the number of nursing assistants the facility employs and what the turnover rate is.
- She should avoid asking questions about pay and benefits until after the job offer has been made.

Forms to bring to a job interview
When going to an interview, a prospective nursing assistant should be prepared.

- She should have a copy of the questions that she plans to ask during the interview.
- She should bring a copy of her resume, preferably printed on fine-quality paper stock.
- She should have a copy of her references, in case the prospective employer wants to check them.
- She should also have any forms that the employer may have requested.
-

All of these things should be kept together using a paperclip and stored in a folder to keep them neat.

Work ethic

Work ethic describes how a person works. If a person has a strong work ethic, it means she works hard at her assigned duties.

- A nursing assistant with a strong work ethic endeavors to complete her assigned tasks in a timely manner, to the best of her ability.
- She works well in a team situation.
- She behaves in a manner that is courteous and accommodating.
- She is punctual, both arriving at work on time and performing tasks at the appointed time.
- A person with a strong work ethic is also reliable, meaning she can be counted on to perform her assigned tasks well without requiring supervision from her charge nurse.

Nursing assistant dress while on duty

Part of behaving in a professional manner is dressing appropriately. Most facilities have a dress code that all employees should follow.

- The nursing assistant should wear scrubs that follow the dress code.
- The scrubs should be clean and well mended.
- Though the scrubs need not be pressed, they should be free of wrinkles.
- Her shoes should be clean and comfortable.
- The nursing assistant should avoid shoes with high heels or open toes.
- The nursing assistant should also wear minimal jewelry and avoid long necklaces, dangling earrings, and rings.
- She should avoid fragrances and perfumes.
- The nursing assistant should keep her nails trimmed and should avoid wearing nail polish or acrylic nails to work.

Responsibilities of a nursing assistant

The nursing assistant's primary responsibility is to care for the patient's basic needs.

- She should see to the patient's nutritional needs by distributing the meal trays and feeding the patient if necessary.
- She should also aid the patient in exercising.
- Whenever necessary, the nursing assistant will aid the patient with elimination and hygiene needs.
- The nursing assistant may be responsible for checking vital signs, answering call lights, and reporting any changes to the charge nurse.
- There may also be other tasks that will be the nursing assistant's responsibility, and these tasks will be detailed by the health care facility.

Maintaining good interpersonal relationships

Good interpersonal relationships are the key to a group of people working as a team. This is necessary in order to provide adequate patient care.

- A nursing assistant can maintain good interpersonal relationships in a number of ways.
- She can behave with a positive attitude.
- She should try to avoid gossiping about coworkers and should avoid openly criticizing them.
- She should perform any tasks assigned to her promptly and should notify the charge nurse if there are any tasks that she is unable to perform during her shift.
- She should also utilize teamwork by regularly offering to provide assistance to others and thanking

them for any assistance provided to her.

Responsibilities in a code situation

In a code situation, it is vital for the health care team to work together in order to provide a positive outcome for the patient.

- Prior to a code, the nursing assistant should be aware of her responsibilities.
- She should know the location of the crash cart in case she is asked to retrieve it and how to activate the code system if she discovers a patient who is unresponsive.
- In a code situation, the nursing assistant's primary role will be to obtain any necessary equipment.
- If she has her CPR certification, the nursing assistant may also provide relief CPR.
- It is important that the nursing assistant listen to any instructions provided to her.
- If the room is crowded, the nursing assistant should leave to make sure it does not remain too crowded but should remain near the door so that she can hear any instructions.

Becoming ill prior to scheduled shift

A nursing assistant should take every precaution to prevent herself from becoming ill.

- If she becomes ill, she should avoid reporting to work, where she could possibly spread her illness to the patient population.
- Most health care facilities have policies regarding sudden illness, and the nursing assistant should make herself aware of these policies.
- Most facilities require the nursing assistant to provide notification of

absence at least two hours prior to the start of her shift.

- It also may be necessary to provide a doctor's excuse if her illness required her to miss multiple days of work.

Scheduling conflict

A nursing assistant should endeavor to make her supervisor aware of any important events so that the facility might work around those events. However, scheduling conflicts do occasionally occur. Most health care facilities do have policies regarding scheduling conflicts, and the nursing assistant should familiarize herself with these policies.

- If a conflict arises, the nursing assistant should talk to her colleagues and try to make arrangements to switch workdays in order to accommodate her schedule.
- If the nursing assistant is unable to find someone to switch with her, she should talk to her supervisor and attempt to make arrangements that can accommodate her schedule.
- Under no circumstances should the nursing assistant not show up for work.

Refusing an assignment

A nursing assistant must have a valid reason to refuse an assignment. There are a number of reasons why she might do so.

- A particular assignment might not be part of a nursing assistant's scope of practice.
- The nursing assistant might feel uncomfortable with the assignment as a result of not knowing how to perform a task or may feel it is unethical or illegal.
- The nursing assistant may refuse an assignment if she feels

performing the task will cause harm to the patient or may place herself in danger if she were to perform that task.

How to refuse an assignment
A nursing assistant should only refuse an assignment if she has a good reason to do so.

- After the assignments have been made, the nursing assistant should talk to the charge nurse privately about her discomfort regarding the assignment.
- She should do so in a calm manner.
- She should explain her concerns and the reason why she is declining the assignment.
- The nursing assistant and the charge nurse should come to an accord regarding the assignment.
- If the nursing assistant and the charge nurse are unable to come to an agreement, the nursing assistant should clearly state that she is declining the assignment.

Patient's family asks to participate in the patient's care

In some cases, a member of the patient's family may express a desire to participate in the patient's care.

- If a family member makes this request, the nursing assistant should notify the charge nurse.
- Ultimately, the decision about allowing the family member to assist with care depends upon the patient as a result of his right to privacy.
- It may be appropriate in some cases, such as if the patient were going home soon and would require assistance at home.
- The nurse should provide instructions to the family member, but the nursing assistant

should be vigilant while the family member is providing care to ensure that it is being properly done.

Delegation

Delegation refers to assigning a task to another person.

- It is within the nurse's scope of practice to assign tasks to the nursing assistant; however, it is not within the nursing assistant's scope of practice to assign tasks to others.
- Though the nursing assistant is responsible for performing the task, it is the responsibility of the nurse to make sure that it is done properly and in a timely manner.
- When assigned a task, the nursing assistant should make sure she understands how to perform that task.
- If she does not know how to do it, the nursing assistant should either ask for instructions in order to perform the task safely or decline the assignment.

Five rights of delegation
It is important for a nursing assistant to understand how a task is delegated in order to know if it is being delegated appropriately. The five rights of delegation can be utilized to determine if the assignment is appropriate.

- The first right refers to the task: whether the task can be delegated to another person or if it is more appropriate for it to be performed by the nurse.
- The second right refers to the circumstance; the nursing assistant should ask herself if the patient is stable enough for the task to be safely performed.

- The third right refers to the right person. The nursing assistant should ask herself if she feels she is able to perform the task appropriately.
- The fourth right refers to directions. The nursing assistant should ask herself if she received adequate instructions regarding the assignment.
- The final right refers to supervision. The nursing assistant should ask herself if she is going to have an appropriate amount of supervision while performing the task.

Practice Test

Practice Questions

1. When performing a bed bath, what temperature should the water be?
    a. 70-80 degrees Fahrenheit
    b. 105-115 degrees Fahrenheit
    c. 130-140 degrees Fahrenheit
    d. 155-165 degrees Fahrenheit

2. Which of the following tasks is NOT completed during a routine bed bath for a diabetic?
    a. Changing the linens
    b. Inspection and cleansing of skin
    c. Perineal care
    d. Nail care

3. How would you classify a pressure sore that has a pink wound bed, but does not extend through the full thickness of the skin?
    a. Stage I
    b. Stage II
    c. Stage III
    d. Stage IV

4. A patient is scheduled for surgery later in the day. What type of food would you expect on his breakfast tray?
    a. No tray – the patient is NPO
    b. Jell-O and chicken broth
    c. Scrambled eggs
    d. French toast and fruit

5. How can a CNA help prevent the development of pressure sores?
    a. Turning the patient every four hours
    b. Providing a full bed bath three times a day
    c. Doing partial baths every time a patient soils herself
    d. Reducing the amount of fluids the patient drinks to minimize incontinence

6. When is it acceptable for a CNA to wash her hands using an alcohol-based hand sanitizer instead of soap and water?
    a. Before eating
    b. After performing peri care on a patient
    c. After using the bathroom
    d. Between checking on patients

7. A CNA is providing care for a patient on contact precautions. What type of personal protective equipment should she be using?
    a. Respirator
    b. Mask
    c. Gown
    d. All of the above

8. Before entering a patient's room, personal protective equipment (PPE) should be put on in which order?
    a. Gown, mask, gloves
    b. Gown, gloves, mask
    c. Mask, gown, gloves
    d. Mask, gloves, gown

9. When changing linens in an isolation room, which of the following is an appropriate measure to prevent contamination of clean materials?
    a. Placing dirty linens in a plastic bag inside of the patient's room, and then putting the plastic bag into a bag outside of the room that is held open by a second CNA
    b. Shaking out soiled linens to remove solid material before washing
    c. Piling soiled linens outside of the dirty utility room to avoid mixing them with non-contaminated linens
    d. Moving the soiled linens to the dirty utility room before hand washing

10. Which of the following items requires cleaning with a disinfectant prior to use?
    a. Stethoscope
    b. Scalpel
    c. Thermometer
    d. Blood pressure cuff

11. What is the proper term for an infection that is transmitted during a medical procedure?
    a. Droplet
    b. Iatrogenic
    c. Direct oral contact
    d. Fecal-oral transmission

12. For a patient on fall precautions, what is the minimum number of side rails that should be raised while the patient is in bed?
    a. 1
    b. 2
    c. 3
    d. 4

13. Before transferring a patient from the bed to a wheelchair, what is the very first thing the CNA should do?
    a. Place her arms under the patient's axilla and assist her to a standing position.
    b. Assist the patient to a sitting position.
    c. Allow the patient to dangle her legs for a few minutes before standing.
    d. Ensure the wheels on both the wheelchair and the bed are locked.

14. What type of assistance would be required for an elderly woman who fell recently, but is still able to ambulate?
    a. Stand by assistance
    b. Minimum assistance
    c. Contact guard assistance
    d. Maximum assistance

15. Which technique is MOST appropriate for a patient with both poor upper body and lower body strength?
    a. Four-point technique
    b. Three-point technique
    c. Swing-to method
    d. Swing-through method

16. A CNA encounters a small fire in a patient's room. The room is empty. What is her first priority?
    a. Rescue patients in the neighboring rooms.
    b. Activate the fire alarm.
    c. Close all fire doors.
    d. Grab a fire extinguisher and attempt to extinguish the fire.

17. Which of the following procedures is NOT appropriate for a patient who has been ordered to be placed in restraints?
    a. Offer toileting and water every one to two hours.
    b. Check the patient at least every 30 minutes to ensure there is proper circulation where the restraints are applied.
    c. Tie the restraints directly to the bed frame.
    d. Tie the restraints directly to the side rails.

18. How should a CNA clean an indwelling catheter?
    a. By using a gentle back and forth motion
    b. By using a circular motion towards the body
    c. By using a circular motion away from the body
    d. By using an up and down motion

19. Before taking a meal tray into a patient's room, what should a CNA do?
    a. Record the amount of food/liquids on the intake/output form.
    b. Assess a patient's ability to swallow properly.
    c. Put on gloves.
    d. Ensure that the correct food is on the tray.

20. If a CNA notices that a patient appears to be having difficulty swallowing, what should she do?
    a. Notify the nurse immediately.
    b. Mash up the food and continue feeding the patient.
    c. Give the patient smaller amounts of food with each bite.
    d. Nothing; the doctor checked the patient's swallowing already.

21. How often should anti-embolism stockings be removed?
    a. Every 4 hours
    b. Every 8 hours
    c. Every 12 hours
    d. Every 24 hours

22. There is a note on a patient's chart that she should be placed in the Sim's position. How should the patient be positioned?
    a. Lying on the stomach with the head turned to the side
    b. On her back with the head of the bed raised to a 90 degree angle
    c. On her back with the head of the bed raised to a 45 degree angle
    d. On her left side with the top leg flexed and supported by a pillow

23. What is the first step for a CNA who is about to put on sterile gloves?
    a. Use the dominant hand to grasp the glove at the cuff and slide it on to the non-dominant hand.
    b. Use the non-dominant hand to grasp the glove under the cuff and slide it on to the dominant hand.
    c. Wash and dry hands thoroughly.
    d. Put on gloves to open the packaging.

24. Which of the following is a measurement of the pressure in a patient's heart during contraction?
    a. Systolic blood pressure
    b. Diastolic blood pressure
    c. Apical pulse
    d. Pulse oximetry

25. Which of the following abnormal vital signs should be immediately reported to the nurse?
    a. Oral temperature of 99.2 degrees
    b. Respiratory rate of 5
    c. Blood pressure of 126/72
    d. Pulse rate of 59

26. Which fluids should be included in the measurement of a patient's intake?
    a. 8 oz. of milk
    b. 250 mL of intravenous fluid
    c. 6 oz. of Jell-O
    d. All of the above

27. What is the first thing a CNA should do when measuring a patient's height and weight?
    a. Wash her hands.
    b. Verify the patient's identity by inspecting her armband.
    c. Allow the patient's legs to dangle for a few moments before allowing her to stand up.
    d. Assist the patient with ambulation to the scale.

28. Which of the following is an example of subjective data?
    a. The patient has a pulse rate of 88 bpm.
    b. The patient states that she has a pain level of 8.
    c. The CNA notes that the patient has flushed cheeks.
    d. The CNA notes that the patient has cloudy urine.

29. While completing her documentation, a CNA notices that she made a mistake while writing in a patient's blood pressure. How should she correct the notation?
    a. Use correction fluid to cover the mistake.
    b. Scribble out the incorrect number and write the correct number next to it.
    c. Draw a single line through the incorrect notation, and write "error," along with her initials. The correct number should be written next to it.
    d. Erase the incorrect notation; documentation is always completed using a pencil.

30. A patient with which of the following conditions is MOST at risk for dehydration?
    a. Diarrhea
    b. Liver disease
    c. Heart disease
    d. Pneumonia

31. When caring for a patient with diarrhea, which of the following should be recorded in the patient's chart?
    a. Odor of the stool
    b. Types and amounts of fluids the patient is drinking
    c. Number of stools
    d. All of the above

32. How often should a patient who is lying on an egg crate or an inflatable mattress be turned?
    a. Never – patients shouldn't be turned when they are lying on inflatable mattresses.
    b. Every 12 hours
    c. Every 6 hours
    d. Every 2 hours

33. Which of the following is NOT an intervention a CNA can use to manage edema?
    a. Elevate the affected extremity.
    b. Use ice or a cold pack to reduce swelling.
    c. Massage the affected extremity using lotion.
    d. Encourage activity or use range of motion exercises.

34. A patient with a shuffling gait, difficulty swallowing and speaking, and short-term memory loss MOST likely has:
    a. Alzheimer's disease
    b. dementia
    c. Parkinson's disease
    d. sundowner's syndrome

35. A CNA is caring for a patient with Sundowner's syndrome. Which of the following symptoms should he be especially aware of?
   a. Worsening confusion at night
   b. Risk for falls
   c. Aggression
   d. Difficulty swallowing

36. What is one technique a CNA can use to help a patient with aphasia?
   a. Providing a time limit for the patient to respond
   b. Speaking for the patient
   c. Using a picture or letter board
   d. Giving the patient a pen

37. A CNA is caring for a patient who is becoming agitated. How should she speak to the patient?
   a. In an assertive and confident manner
   b. Not at all; the patient's family members or other staff should interact with the patient.
   c. She should not acknowledge the inappropriate behavior and carry on as normal.
   d. Calmly and clearly, while attempting to determine why the patient is agitated

38. Hospice care is appropriate for patients who:
   a. are expected to live less than three months.
   b. are expected to live less than six months.
   c. are actively dying.
   d. have been diagnosed with a terminal disease, regardless of their clinical condition.

39. Which of the following answer choices correctly lists the five stages of grief in order of their expected occurrence?
   a. Denial, anger, bargaining, depression, acceptance
   b. Anger, denial, depression, bargaining, acceptance
   c. Depression, denial, anger, bargaining, acceptance
   d. Bargaining, denial, anger, depression, acceptance

40. Unless otherwise ordered, how often should a CNA record the vital signs of a patient who is actively dying? The patient has a signed DNR order in place.
   a. Every 5 minutes
   b. Every 15 minutes
   c. Every hour
   d. Never

41. While you are caring for a Buddhist patient, he mentions an upcoming fast day when he can only eat at predetermined times during the day. What is an appropriate response?
   a. Acknowledge his beliefs but explain that you can't make any changes to the facility's dining times.
   b. Suggest that his family bring some food from home.
   c. Speak with him to determine what his needs will be that day and coordinate with the dining and food team.
   d. Apologize for not being able to help him that day.

42. When caring for a Jewish patient who observes the Kosher laws, the CNA notices his dinner plate has a dish with pork in it. What should the CNA do?
    a. Bring him the food tray and see if he requests a change.
    b. Call the dining/food department to order a new tray, and explain the delay to the patient.
    c. Remove the pork from his plate and serve him the tray.
    d. Switch trays with another patient.

43. What needs are found on the bottom level of Maslow's pyramid?
    a. Physiological
    b. Safety/security
    c. Love and belonging
    d. Self-esteem

44. A CNA needs to speak with a patient about the quality and amount of stool he passed that day. How can the CNA help the patient feel more comfortable about disclosing the needed information?
    a. Ask the patient in his room when visitors are present.
    b. Ask the patient in the privacy of his room in a quiet tone.
    c. Ask the patient in an indirect way and hope the patient understands what the CNA is trying to ask.
    d. Ask the patient closed-ended questions.

45. A patient states that she is depressed. Which of the following responses by the CNA involves the use of reflection?
    a. I'm sorry that you're feeling depressed.
    b. Why are you feeling depressed? Your recovery is moving along well.
    c. Do you want to speak with someone about this?
    d. You feel depressed?

46. A CNA is stocking shelves outside a patient's room when the call bell rings. The CNA is not responsible for the patient's care that day. How should the CNA respond?
    a. Ignoring the call bell until the patient's assigned CNA responds
    b. Getting the assigned CNA to check on the patient
    c. Checking on the patient right away to see what she needs
    d. Checking on the patient after stocking the shelves

47. A patient has rung the call bell for the sixth time during the first two hours of a CNA's shift. How should she respond?
    a. Ignore the bell.
    b. Call the nurse manager.
    c. Remove the bell from the patient's reach.
    d. Reassure the patient she will be checked on frequently.

48. A CNA has been assigned to care for a ventilated patient, which she has never done before. How should she handle the situation?

    a. Notify the nurse manager that she is not sure how to care for the patient, and request additional instructions or training materials.

    b. Do the best she can while caring for the patient.

    c. Speak with the other CNAs to find out what additional care is needed for the patient.

    d. Request to switch patients with another CNA.

49. A CNA has to ask a sensitive question to a patient who doesn't speak English. How should she ask the question?

    a. Using the patient's family to translate

    b. Calling the hospital's official translation service

    c. Gesturing to the patient in the hope she will understand

    d. Looking up relevant words on the Internet before speaking with the patient

50. A patient's family asks how he is doing after his scheduled MRI. How should the CNA respond?

    a. He had an MRI today?

    b. His MRI results are back. Everything is normal.

    c. He seems to be in good spirits. Let me see if he's ready to visit with you and I'll find his nurse to talk to you about the results.

    d. Good. He should be ready to go home soon.

51. HIPAA guarantees a patient's right to:

    a. confidentiality.

    b. informed consent.

    c. see their chart.

    d. continuity of care.

52. A patient has a few questions about the consent forms she signed for a scheduled invasive procedure. How should the CNA respond?

    a. Answer the questions to the best of her ability.

    b. Tell the patient that she will ask the nurse to contact the doctor.

    c. Tell the patient that she will have plenty of time to ask the doctor before the procedure.

    d. Remind the patient that she signed the consent and that the procedure has already been scheduled.

53. A family member gives a copy of a patient's advanced directives to a CNA. The patient is scheduled for a minor procedure the next day. Which of the following is an appropriate response?

    a. Tell them to hold onto the copies until and unless they are needed.

    b. Tell the family that they are not necessary because the patient is having a minor surgical procedure.

    c. Put the copy in the chart.

    d. Immediately notify the nurse that the family has advanced directives for the patient.

54. A patient is refusing to be turned and it has been several hours since he was last turned. The patient is alert and oriented. How should the CNA respond?
    a. Turn him anyway; he needs it to prevent skin breakdown.
    b. Inform him that she will tell the doctor he is refusing care so he can go home.
    c. Inform him of the associated risks, and then respect his decision if he still does not want to be turned.
    d. Tell him whatever is necessary to obtain his consent to be turned.

55. Which of the following would NOT be included in a list of patient responsibilities?
    a. Honesty
    b. Polite and respectful behavior
    c. Maintain all personal property
    d. Compliance with treatment plan

56. A nurse asks a CNA to give Tylenol to a patient who has a headache. The nurse is very busy with another critical patient. What should the CNA do?
    a. Administer the Tylenol; the nurse did the assessment and delegated this task to her.
    b. Refuse to give the patient any medication – it is not within her scope of practice.
    c. Find the Tylenol and repeat the order – including the patient's name, room number, and instructions – back to the nurse to confirm her directions.
    d. Ask another nurse to give the medication.

57. While in an elevator, another CNA asks you about the MRI results for the patient in room 307. The CNA cared for the patient while on another unit. What is an appropriate response?
    a. Refuse to answer the question; the CNA is no longer an active member of the patient's health care team.
    b. Answer the question fully and honestly.
    c. Answer the question without using any identifying information so the others in the elevator won't know who you are talking about.
    d. Wait until the other people exit the elevator to answer the question.

58. A patient who was injured while committing a criminal act has a right to treatment under which of the following patient rights?
    a. Right to freedom of choice
    b. Right to respectful care
    c. Right to continuity of care
    d. Right of refusal

59. A patient demands to see his medical chart. The CNA should:
    a. give the patient his chart and leave the room to give him privacy.
    b. give the patient the chart and stay in the room to ensure he doesn't make any changes.
    c. make photocopies of the chart and give them to the patient.
    d. inform him that he will need to notify the medical records department to make arrangements.

60. A doctor writes a DNR order to:
    a. prevent any care from being provided to a patient.
    b. explain the care the doctor feels would most benefit a patient.
    c. explain what type of emergency care a patient wishes to have.
    d. discharge a patient into hospice care.

61. If a patient refuses a treatment and the CNA attempts to perform it anyway, what could the CNA be charged with?
    a. Assault
    b. Battery
    c. Either A or B
    d. Neither A nor B

62. A CNA who forgets to lock the wheels on a wheelchair (which results in a subsequent fall) could be charged with:
    a. assault.
    b. battery.
    c. malpractice.
    d. negligence.

63. If a CNA observes the nursing supervisor acting in a negligent way, what should she do?
    a. Speak with the doctor in charge of the patient.
    b. Follow the institution's chain of command to determine who to report the behavior to.
    c. Go to the institution's president of nursing to report the behavior.
    d. Confront the nursing supervisor directly.

64. If a CNA begins to suspect that a patient is being abused by a family member, what should she do?
    a. Report it to the charge nurse.
    b. Report it to the police.
    c. Ignore it because the nurse and doctor probably suspect it too.
    d. Confront the suspected abuser.

65. Who is the most important member of the health care team?
    a. The nurse
    b. The patient
    c. The physician
    d. The CNA

66. What is the minimum number of hours of continuing education that a CNA should complete each year?
    a. 6
    b. 12
    c. 20
    d. 50

67. What is the BEST way for a CNA to assist during a code?
   a. Administer emergency medications according to the physician's instructions.
   b. Document the events.
   c. Speak with the family and answer their questions about what is happening.
   d. Retrieve emergency equipment, including the code cart or intubation box, and carry out other assigned tasks that fall within a CNA's scope of practice.

68. A patient's daughter is requesting to perform morning care for her mother. The patient is okay with the request, and it has been cleared with the charge nurse. What should the CNA do?
   a. Refuse to let the daughter assist.
   b. Allow her to perform the morning care and leave the room to provide privacy.
   c. Allow her to assist with morning care, but stay in the room to ensure it is being done correctly.
   d. Request that the nurse supervise the patient's daughter.

69. When the CNA is informed of an admission, what is her responsibility?
   a. Prepare the room, including the linens, gowns, and other necessary equipment.
   b. Complete the admissions interview.
   c. Make sure the patient's medications have been received from the pharmacy and are correct.
   d. Coordinate the patient's care with the rest of the treatment team.

70. Which of the following is NOT a reason for a CNA to refuse an assignment?
   a. The CNA feels the task is unethical.
   b. Performing the task would cause harm to the CNA.
   c. The CNA had a serious disagreement with the patient's family the day before.
   d. The assignment is outside the CNA's scope of practice.

Answers and Explanations

1. B: Water for a bed bath should be heated up to approximately 105 to 115 degrees Fahrenheit. Any cooler and the water will cool off too much before the end of the bath, chilling the patient. Any warmer and the water will be too hot, and could potentially burn the patient. Filling the basin should be the last thing you do; gather all other supplies first to minimize the cooling of the water. If you don't have a thermometer to measure the water temperature, make sure it is comfortably warm against your elbow or inner arm.

2. D: You should check with your institution's policies on nail care, but generally speaking, a CNA should not provide nail care to a diabetic patient. Diabetics have impaired circulation to their extremities, which can delay healing and even cause severe damage if the skin is injured. For that reason, only a physician, podiatrist, or other specially trained clinician should perform nail care on a diabetic. Performing perineal care, changing the linens, and inspecting the skin should be done during every full bed bath, usually as part of morning care.

3. B: A stage I pressure sore would appear as a reddened area that does not blanch (turn white) when pressed. A stage II pressure sore involves a partial breakdown of the upper layer of skin, but does not extend all the way through the skin. A stage II pressure ulcer may look like a blister. Stage III and stage IV ulcers extend all the way through the skin. You may see the underlying subcutaneous fat in a stage III ulcer, whereas a stage IV may proceed all the way down to the muscles, tendons, or bones. Make sure to report any skin redness to the nurse so that the skin can be thoroughly assessed.

4. A: A patient who is about to undergo surgery or another procedure requiring an anesthetic should be NPO for a minimum of eight hours before the procedure. If the patient receives a tray, you should double check with the nurse before serving the patient his breakfast. If a procedure is scheduled for later in the day, the anesthesiologist may be okay with the patient eating breakfast.

5. C: A patient who is bedbound or spends a majority of the day lying or sitting down is at risk for developing pressure sores. Preventing pressure sores requires multiple interventions, including: turning the patient every two hours, doing a full bed bath once a day and partial bed baths throughout the day as necessary if the patient is incontinent (partial baths should be done whenever a patient soils himself), increasing the protein content of food, and making sure the patient is hydrated. It is not appropriate to do a full bed bath twice a day. Withholding fluids to prevent incontinence is also inappropriate.

6. D: Alcohol-based sanitizers are a great tool to avoid the comparatively time-consuming process of hand washing, and are appropriate in certain situations. The CNA should wash her hands with soap and water before eating, after using the bathroom, after performing a procedure that involves contact with bodily fluids (such as peri care), and when her hands are visibly soiled. She should also wash her hands periodically throughout the day to remove the buildup of alcohol on the hands. It is perfectly acceptable to use an alcohol-based sanitizer between checking on patients, especially if the CNA is not performing care.

7. C: If a patient is on contact precautions the caretaker must wear a gown and gloves. Using a mask or respirator is not necessary unless the patient is on droplet or airborne precautions.

8. A: When entering the room of a patient on isolation precautions, the CNA should put on the gown first, with the opening in the back. After tying the gown closed at the neck and around the waist, the mask should be put on next. Lastly, the CNA should put on her gloves, ensuring that the cuff of the gloves is covering the cuff of the gown. When leaving the room, the PPE should be removed in the reverse order: gloves, mask, and gown.

9. A: Anything in the patient's room is considered "contaminated," so when you place the soiled linens into the plastic linen bag, that bag is considered contaminated. The CNA should ask a colleague to hold a second bag open at the doorway and place the contaminated linen bag in it. The second CNA can then put the bag on the floor outside of the room until the first CNA is ready to wash her hands and bring it to the dirty utility room. The soiled linens should never be shaken out because of the risk of contaminating other nearby items.

10. C: Items that require cleaning with a disinfectant are ones that come into contact with a patient's mucus membranes but don't puncture the skin. Thermometers and respiratory equipment are good examples of items that should be disinfected but don't require sterilization. Items such as scalpels that penetrate the skin should be sterilized between patients because of the high risk of contamination. Items such as stethoscopes and blood pressure cuffs that just touch the skin can be cleaned with a mild detergent between uses.

11. B: An infection that is transmitted during a medical procedure is called iatrogenic. Droplet transmission is when bacteria or viruses are released in droplets when a person sneezes or coughs. Direct oral contact is transmission between people when there is direct oral contact, such as kissing or sharing a drinking cup. Fecal-oral contamination is exactly what it sounds like: fecal material contaminates food, usually through poor hand washing or poor food preparation techniques.

12. B: A minimum of two bed rails should be raised when the patient is in bed. Raising four side rails is considered a restraint, and should not be done unless directly ordered by the physician. One raised bed rail leaves an entire side of the bed without any boundaries.

13. D: The very first thing that should be done before transferring a patient is to make sure that the wheels on both the wheelchair and the bed are locked. This prevents falls by preventing movement of the bed or wheelchair as the patient is being transferred. Once the CNA has verified that the wheels are locked, she can help the patient to sit up and allow her to dangle her legs for a few moments. Then, she can help the patient stand up and slide into the wheelchair.

14. C: An elderly woman who has fallen previously is at risk for falling again. However, she is still ambulatory, so the CNA should be within an arm's reach in case the patient becomes unsteady or falls again. This is known as contact guard assistance. Stand by assistance and maximum assistance are inappropriate because they provide too little and too much support, respectively.

15. A: Four-point technique is a great method of crutch walking for patients who have poor upper and lower body strength because it balances out the patient's weight on both arms

and the alternating legs. Three-point, swing-to, and swing-through methods are all great for a patient who has good upper body strength because these gaits depend primarily on the arms to keep the patient upright.

16. B: This question can be answered using the acronym R.A.C.E. (rescue, activate alarm, confine the fire, evacuate/extinguish). The CNA should first rescue patients in imminent danger. Because the room is empty, her first priority should be to pull the fire alarm. If the fire is small and contained, she could try to extinguish the fire herself with a fire extinguisher using the P.A.S.S. method (pull the pin, aim at the base of the fire, and sweep side to side). If not, she should start closing fire doors and rescuing patients in neighboring rooms if necessary.

17. D: Whenever a patient is placed in restraints, the CNA should make sure there is an up-to-date order from the physician (within the last 24 hours). The patient should be offered the opportunity to use the bathroom or have a glass of water or food at least every one to two hours. The restraints should be checked at least every thirty minutes to make sure they are not too tight or cutting off circulation to the patient's limbs. The ties should be quick-release knots and the restraints should be tied directly to the bed frame. Restraints should never be tied to the side rails in case they inadvertently fall, which could cause injury to the patient.

18. C: A patient with an indwelling catheter has a higher risk of contracting a urinary tract infection, and so catheter and perineal care is very important. The catheter should be assessed and cleaned frequently. After putting on gloves and explaining what you are going to do, you should use warm water to gently clean the urethra and, using a circular motion away from the body, the catheter. The CNA should never clean upwards or use a back and forth motion because of the potential to introduce bacteria into the urethra. Make sure to dry the catheter and patient, check to make sure there are no kinks in the tubing, and then hang the bag from the bed frame.

19. D: Before taking a meal tray into a patient's room, the CNA should ensure that the tray is labeled with the correct name, room number, and diet. Once she has delivered all of the trays, the CNA can go back and assist patients who need help eating. Ability to swallow should be assessed each time a patient is eating. The CNA should always be alert for signs that the patient isn't swallowing properly. As she is collecting the used food trays, the CNA should document the intake for each patient. This is the best time to see what each patient actually ate.

20. A: Because of the serious risk of aspiration and its complications, the CNA should never continue feeding food to a patient with a suspected swallowing issue. She should immediately stop feeding the patient and notify the nurse. The nurse can inform the doctor and arrange for a swallowing study if necessary, or even change the patient's diet to include soft foods or purées only.

21. B: Anti-embolism stockings should be removed once every eight hours to ensure proper circulation and let the skin breathe. When removing the stockings, the CNA should assess the skin to make sure there are no rashes, skin breakdown, or other concerns. She should also check on the patient's toes to assess blood flow while the stockings are on. If the patient

complains of numbness, tingling, or discomfort when wearing the stockings, it should be brought to the nurse's attention immediately.

22. D: Sim's position is when a patient is lying on her side with the top leg flexed towards the chest. Choice A, on her stomach, is called the prone position. Choice B, with the head of the bed raised to a 90 degree angle, is called the High Fowler's position. Choice C, on her back with the head of the bed raised to 45 degrees, is called the Semi-Fowler's position.

23. C: When putting on sterile gloves, the CNA should first wash and dry her hands thoroughly. Then, she should open the packaging, taking care not to touch anything inside. Next, she should pick up the glove for the dominant hand at the cuff using her non-dominant hand and slide it onto the dominant hand. Finally, using the gloved hand, she should pick up the second glove beneath the cuff and slide it onto the non-dominant hand. Once both gloves are on, she can then make adjustments to the fit, taking care to avoid touching anything unsterile.

24. A: Systolic blood pressure, or the top number of the patient's blood pressure, looks at the pressure in the patient's heart during contraction. Diastolic blood pressure, or the lower number, looks at the pressure in the heart during rest. The pulse measures the number of cardiac contractions per minute. Pulse oximetry measures the amount of oxygen in the blood.

25. B: Choices A and D are slightly abnormal and should be reported to the nurse, although it is not necessary to do this immediately. A blood pressure of 126/72 is technically considered abnormal, but can probably be largely attributed to the stress of being in the hospital. It is nothing to be overly concerned about. A respiratory rate of five breaths per minute is very slow, and can indicate impending respiratory failure. The CNA should notify the nurse immediately.

26. D: All of the choices are liquids or melt at room temperature (Jell-O), and should be included in the measurement of a patient's intake. The CNA should also measure the amount of tube feeding (including what is used to flush the tube) and other IV medications or fluids. Total intake should be in ccs or mLs (depending on your institution's policies) and recorded every 24 hours.

27. A: Whenever a CNA enters a patient's room to initiate care or perform a task, she should wash her hands, introduce herself to the patient, and explain what she is going to do. Next, she should identify the patient using the patient's armband and two identifiers. Finally, she can perform the task she came in to do, which in this case is measuring the patient's height and weight.

28. B: Subjective data is anything the patient notes or feels, such as her pain level. Objective data is information that can be measured (such as vital signs) or observed by another person (such as the patient having cloudy urine or flushed cheeks).

29. C: Making documentation errors is common. However, the CNA must understand how to deal with these errors. She should never use correction fluid or scribble out the error so it is illegible. A pencil should never be used for documentation. When an error is made, simply

draw a single line through the mistake and place the correction, the word "error," and your initials next to it.

30. A: A patient with diarrhea is at a high risk for dehydration, so all complaints from the patient and direct observations of diarrhea should be reported to the nurse. Signs of dehydration include dry mucus membranes, weakness, and thirst. The CNA may also observe dark urine or sunken eyes. As long as it's not contraindicated, the CNA should encourage the patient to drink extra water to help replace the lost fluids.

31. D: When caring for a patient with diarrhea, it is important to note all of the information in the answer choices in the patient's chart, as it can be vitally important to the care and treatment plan for the patient. Additionally, the doctor will need the information to gauge the severity of the diarrhea and dehydration. The CNA should also note how much fluid is passed with each stool and how often the patient is having episodes of diarrhea.

32. D: Unless the patient is on a special bed that is designed to be used without turning, the patient should always be turned every two hours. Simply adding an egg crate or inflatable mattress to the existing bed is not enough to eliminate or reduce the need to turn the patient. An egg crate can help reduce the pressure on the patient's skin and bony prominences, but the patient should still be turned every two hours.

33. B: True edema is usually a result of poor circulation, so using an ice or cold pack would be of little use in managing it. Useful interventions help stimulate blood flow and blood return. Elevating the extremity will help promote lymphatic drainage and venous return to minimize edema. Movement through ambulation, massage, or range of motion exercises are also great ways to treat and minimize edema.

34. C: All of these symptoms are signs of Parkinson's disease. Alzheimer's disease, dementia, and Sundowner's syndrome all produce similar symptoms, which include confusion, agitation, and wandering. A shuffling gait, though, is the hallmark symptom of Parkinson's disease. A patient with Parkinson's needs special help with ambulation because their gait is so unsteady, and with eating because they frequently have difficulty swallowing their food.

35. A: Patients with Sundowner's syndrome typically have worsening confusion at night. They may become agitated and wander off the unit. During the day, patients with Sundowner's typically aren't as confused. Possible interventions include checking on and reorienting the patient frequently, and preventing day time sleep so that it is easier for the patient to sleep at night. A patient with Sundowner's may also be at risk for falls or aggression or have difficulty swallowing, but these symptoms are secondary to the confusion they experience at night.

36. C: Aphasia is an acquired inability to understand language and express oneself through speech. Patients with aphasia have different levels of ability, and should be approached with patience. Setting a time limit and speaking for the patient are not productive or helpful in terms of helping the patient relearn these skills. A pen and paper may be helpful in some situations, but many patients aren't able to read or write as a result of their aphasia. A picture or letter board is a universal method of communication, and offers an easy way to communicate because it is so simple to use.

37. D: Patients may become agitated for any number of reasons. They might be in pain or be uncomfortable. They could be hungry, thirsty, have to go to the bathroom, or even be bored or scared. Understanding what is causing someone's agitation is the best way to relieve it. The CNA should continue to interact with the patient in a calm, clear, and professional manner. She may need to set boundaries as necessary, especially if the behavior persists.

38. B: Hospice care is appropriate for patients who are expected to live less than six months. Patients who are transferred into hospice care typically sign a DNR order and are treated using pain relief measures.

39. A: The first stage of grief is denial that the event happened or is going to happen. Following that is anger at the situation or people involved. Next is bargaining, in which the sufferer bargains with God (I'll do…… if you make this go away). Depression follows as the person starts to deal with their grief. Finally, the patient begins to accept what has happened and can start to move forward. It's important to keep in mind that not everyone goes through the same steps in a linear and straightforward manner. It's not uncommon for someone to progress through one stage quickly and then get held up at a subsequent stage or even regress back to a prior stage.

40. D: Generally speaking, the CNA should never record the vital signs of a patient with a DNR order in place who is actively dying. The clinical staff, including the CNA, should do everything in their power to make the patient and their family comfortable. The family may want the extra time with their loved one without being interrupted. Additionally, the act of having their vital signs taken may cause pain or discomfort for the patient, both of which should be avoided if possible. If, however, the physician has ordered otherwise, the CNA should defer to the wishes of the physician and nurse.

41. C: A patient's religion plays a huge role in how well a patient is able to heal and cope with their disease. The CNA should advocate for her patient and arrange for meals to be sent up at the designated times. She could also coordinate with the nurse and other staff members to ensure continuity. Having his family bring food from home may be one possibility, but the CNA should first try to make arrangements with the dining department.

42. B: Kosher dietary laws are strict guidelines that people who belong to the Jewish faith must follow. The CNA should be sensitive to that and arrange for another tray to be sent up from the dining department. It is not appropriate to simply remove the pork from the patient's tray or wait until the patient requests a change. The CNA should not switch his tray with another patient's. Each tray is specially prepared based on patients' nutritional needs and allergies.

43. A: Physiological needs must be met first, and are therefore at the bottom of the pyramid. These needs include food, water, sex, and oxygen. The next level is the need for safety and security. This isn't restricted to just physical security, but also the safety of one's family, morals, finances, employment, and property. Love and belonging (usually to a group such as a family or friends) is the next level. The final two levels are self-esteem (encompassing self-confidence and achievement) followed by self-actualization, which includes creativity, spontaneity, and morality.

44. B: When speaking with a patient about sensitive topics, it can be helpful to ask the patient when he is alone and use a quiet, sensitive tone. The CNA should be direct, however, and avoid using clichés or euphemisms. It can also be helpful to use open-ended questions, which gives patients the opportunity to answer for themselves.

45. D: Reflection is the process of listening to what patients say and reflecting it back to them, giving them an opportunity to further explain what they meant. This is the technique used in Choice d. Choice A is an example of showing empathy. Choice B is not helpful for the patient; they may be feeling depressed for reasons that are entirely unrelated to their illness. The response is not sensitive to the patient's needs. Choice C may be appropriate, but shuts down the conversation and the relationship between the patient and the CNA.

46. C: Because of the potential for a patient emergency, it is never appropriate for a CNA to ignore a call bell. She should respond to the bell and see if she is able to assist the patient. Stocking the shelves is not a priority, especially when it comes to patient care. It may be necessary for the CNA to get the assigned aid to help with patient care, but she should verify that nothing urgent is needed first.

47. D: The CNA should never ignore a patient's call bell because it could potentially alert the staff to a dangerous situation. That doesn't mean, however, that the patient has a right to abuse the staff and call bell system. The CNA should establish clear boundaries and expectations about when it is okay to use the call bell. She should also understand that it is quite likely that the patient is anxious or lonely, and should agree to check on her at established intervals. This may help alleviate some of the anxiety. The nurse manager may need to get involved if the above interventions aren't successful.

48. A: The CNA should never take on a patient or task that she does not feel sufficiently trained to handle or comfortable with. She should immediately speak privately with the nurse manager to request additional instructions or training. The CNA should never "just do the best she can" because of the potential for serious complications. Colleagues may be an additional source of information, but the nurse manager should be immediately made aware of the situation, and should be the primary point of contact for the CNA.

49. B: When a sensitive topic is involved, the CNA should utilize the hospital's translation system. This can help the patient feel more comfortable and answer the question more appropriately and accurately. Family members are a good source of assistance for routine tasks and matters that don't involve sensitive topics. Gesturing to the patient in the hope she will understand the question is not a great technique because it can easily lead to misunderstanding. Looking up words on the Internet can be helpful, but will not guarantee that either the patient or the CNA will understand what the other is trying to say.

50. C: Unless the family member has a legal document stating that they are the patient's guardian or holds power of attorney, the patient has a right to privacy. Further, the CNA should not give results to any patient or family member. It's fine to say that the patient seems to be feeling well and offer to get the nurse to discuss details about the test.

51. A: HIPAA guarantees a patient's confidentiality and privacy. It also requires healthcare providers to provide patients with a list of policies that have been designed to protect their

privacy. Only providers who are directly caring for someone should have access to their medical chart.

52. B: A CNA should not discuss procedures or what was in the consent forms the patient signed. Only a physician can review and inform a patient of the risks and benefits of having a procedure or treatment. A patient can always withdraw their consent, even if they're about to go into the procedure room. The nurse should notify the physician that the patient has questions so he can arrange to see the patient and discuss her concerns.

53. D: Advanced directives should be promptly placed in the patient's chart and the nurse or physician should be notified. They may need to verify the orders or write new orders for the hospital's order system. Everyone involved in the care of the patient needs to be on the same page and aware of the patient's wishes, even if they are only having a minor procedure.

54. C: A patient has the right to refuse a procedure, even if doing so is not in his best interest. The CNA should explain why frequent turning is important and what may happen if he continues to refuse. Asking what the patient is concerned about or why he doesn't want to be turned can be helpful in identifying solvable problems. If the patient still refuses, the CNA should notify the nurse, who can also speak with the patient and document the incident in the chart.

55. C: All of the choices with the exception of maintenance of personal property are patient responsibilities. Valuable items should be returned to the patient's home or stored with hospital security. Patients should be honest with their caregivers and act in a respectful and appropriate manner. While a patient has the right to refuse treatment, it is expected that they will work with the care team to develop and maintain a mutually acceptable treatment plan.

56. B: A CNA should never administer medication; it's not within her scope of practice. The CNA should go back to the patient and explain that the nurse is with a critical patient and will be with her as soon as possible. Asking another nurse to administer the medication is not an appropriate action because the CNA is then accepting responsibility for delegating the task to another staff member.

57. A: You should refuse to answer the question. The patient has a right to privacy and confidentiality. Even though the colleague cared for the patient in the past, she is not a current, active member of the patient's healthcare team. Therefore, the CNA does not have a right to that information.

58. B: The patient in this situation has a right to respectful care. All patients have the right to receive care, even people injured in the course of committing a crime or those already in the criminal justice system. Patients also have the right to receive care without being discriminated against on the basis of age, gender, nationality, or religion. The right to freedom of choice is the patient's right to have a say in their care plan, and to refuse certain treatments or refuse care altogether.

59. D: A patient absolutely has the right to see his medical chart, but he must follow the procedures put in place by the institution in order to do so. In most cases, the patient will

need to contact the medical records department and submit a formal request in writing. The CNA should not provide copies directly to the patient.

60. C: A DNR order is written for a patient so that the health care team involved in his treatment understands what type of emergency care the patient wishes to have should he become incapacitated. It does not release the physician from providing any care, but simply explains the patient's wishes. For example, the patient may not want to be intubated, but may consent to antibiotics or a feeding tube. In most cases, pain management continues to be an important part of a patient's care, even with a DNR order in place. Often, a DNR order is required for patients entering hospice care, but it is not the only reason why a patient would have such an order.

61. C: A CNA could be charged with assault if she threatens or tries to touch a patient (provide care) without the patient's consent. It does not matter if she actually touches the patient or provides the treatment; the patient just needs to be afraid that she will do it. Battery refers to the actual act of touching the patient in a threatening manner or in a way that the patient has not consented to. In the situation outlined in the question, the CNA could be charged with both assault and/or battery, depending on the specific circumstances surrounding the incident.

62. D: The CNA could be charged with negligence because she performed a task in a way that was inconsistent with her training. Only a professional with advanced training or one who needs to maintain a license, such as a doctor or nurse, can be charged with malpractice. A CNA can't because they only need to maintain a certification, not a license. Assault and battery do not apply because the CNA is not behaving in a threatening manner.

63. B: The CNA should follow the chain of command when determining who to report the behavior to. It is inappropriate to contact the physician in charge of the patient's care because he does not have any authority to deal with this type of nursing situation. It is inappropriate to go directly to the nursing supervisor or president of nursing without following the guidelines set in place by the institution.

64. A: The CNA should immediately report the suspected abuse to the charge nurse so she can determine how best to proceed. It is possible that the suspicions have already been addressed, which is why it is not appropriate to directly report the suspected abuse to the police or confront the potential abuser. The behavior should not be ignored, however, because of the potential for the patient being harmed.

65. B: The most important member of the health care team is the patient. His or her needs—medical, spiritual, and emotional—are the most important. The patient must ultimately consent to and be actively involved in their plan of care. What the physician, nurse, and CNA need, recommend, or want takes a back seat to the needs and wishes of the patient.

66. B: The CNA should complete a minimum of 12 hours of continuing education each year to keep her skills up to date. Additional continuing education hours may be necessary, depending on the skill level and needs of the CNA. Her employer should provide some of the continuing education credits, but it is ultimately the responsibility of the CNA to maintain her certification.

67. D: During a code, the CNA should promptly retrieve emergency equipment or other supplies according to the needs of the physicians and nurses. That may include blood from the blood bank, needles, syringes, etc. Documenting the events and administering medications is the responsibility of the nurse, and is outside the scope of practice of the CNA. The CNA should not answer medical questions from the family, but may be able to provide comfort or support if necessary.

68. C: In cases where the patient will be going home to be cared for by the family, it is definitely appropriate for family members to begin to assist in the patient's care. The CNA should allow the daughter to participate in her mother's care, but should be available to supervise and assist as necessary.

69. A: The CNA should prepare the room, ensuring that linens, personal protective equipment, and other medical supplies are present. The CNA should also help orient the patient to the unit and take vital signs. The nurse should complete the admission interview and assessment and coordinate all aspects of care. This includes contacting the pharmacy and ensuring the correct medications are received.

70. C - A serious disagreement with the patient's family is not a reason to refuse an assignment. The CNA must find a way to work professionally with her patient and the family. If the disagreement begins to interfere with the care the patient is receiving, the CNA should speak with her nurse supervisor about the steps that will need to be taken. The other answer choices are all valid reasons for refusing an assignment.

Secret Key #1 - Time is Your Greatest Enemy

Pace Yourself

Wear a watch. At the beginning of the test, check the time (or start a chronometer on your watch to count the minutes), and check the time after every few questions to make sure you are "on schedule."

If you are forced to speed up, do it efficiently. Usually one or more answer choices can be eliminated without too much difficulty. Above all, don't panic. Don't speed up and just begin guessing at random choices. By pacing yourself, and continually monitoring your progress against your watch, you will always know exactly how far ahead or behind you are with your available time. If you find that you are one minute behind on the test, don't skip one question without spending any time on it, just to catch back up. Take 15 fewer seconds on the next four questions, and after four questions you'll have caught back up. Once you catch back up, you can continue working each problem at your normal pace.

Furthermore, don't dwell on the problems that you were rushed on. If a problem was taking up too much time and you made a hurried guess, it must be difficult. The difficult questions are the ones you are most likely to miss anyway, so it isn't a big loss. It is better to end with more time than you need than to run out of time.

Lastly, sometimes it is beneficial to slow down if you are constantly getting ahead of time. You are always more likely to catch a careless mistake by working more slowly than quickly, and among very high-scoring test takers (those who are likely to have lots of time left over), careless errors affect the score more than mastery of material.

Secret Key #2 - Guessing is not Guesswork

You probably know that guessing is a good idea - unlike other standardized tests, there is no penalty for getting a wrong answer. Even if you have no idea about a question, you still have a 20-25% chance of getting it right.

Most test takers do not understand the impact that proper guessing can have on their score. Unless you score extremely high, guessing will significantly contribute to your final score.

Monkeys Take the Test

What most test takers don't realize is that to insure that 20-25% chance, you have to guess randomly. If you put 20 monkeys in a room to take this test, assuming they answered once per question and behaved themselves, on average they would get 20-25% of the questions correct. Put 20 test takers in the room, and the average will be much lower among guessed questions. Why?

1. The test writers intentionally write deceptive answer choices that "look" right. A test taker has no idea about a question, so picks the "best looking" answer, which is often wrong. The monkey has no idea what looks good and what doesn't, so will consistently be lucky about 20-25% of the time.
2. Test takers will eliminate answer choices from the guessing pool based on a hunch or intuition. Simple but correct answers often get excluded, leaving a 0% chance of being correct. The monkey has no clue, and often gets lucky with the best choice.

This is why the process of elimination endorsed by most test courses is flawed and detrimental to your performance- test takers don't guess, they make an ignorant stab in the dark that is usually worse than random.

$5 Challenge

Let me introduce one of the most valuable ideas of this course- the $5 challenge:

You only mark your "best guess" if you are willing to bet $5 on it.
You only eliminate choices from guessing if you are willing to bet $5 on it.

Why $5? Five dollars is an amount of money that is small yet not insignificant, and can really add up fast (20 questions could cost you $100). Likewise, each answer choice on one question of the test will have a small impact on your overall score, but it can really add up to a lot of points in the end.

The process of elimination IS valuable. The following shows your chance of guessing it right:

If you eliminate wrong answer choices until only this many remain:	Chance of getting it correct:
1	100%
2	50%
3	33%

However, if you accidentally eliminate the right answer or go on a hunch for an incorrect answer, your chances drop dramatically: to 0%. By guessing among all the answer choices, you are GUARANTEED to have a shot at the right answer.

That's why the $5 test is so valuable- if you give up the advantage and safety of a pure guess, it had better be worth the risk.

What we still haven't covered is how to be sure that whatever guess you make is truly random. Here's the easiest way:

Always pick the first answer choice among those remaining.

Such a technique means that you have decided, **before you see a single test question**, exactly how you are going to guess- and since the order of choices tells you nothing about which one is correct, this guessing technique is perfectly random.

This section is not meant to scare you away from making educated guesses or eliminating choices- you just need to define when a choice is worth eliminating. The $5 test, along with a pre-defined random guessing strategy, is the best way to make sure you reap all of the benefits of guessing.

Secret Key #3 - Practice Smarter, Not Harder

Many test takers delay the test preparation process because they dread the awful amounts of practice time they think necessary to succeed on the test. We have refined an effective method that will take you only a fraction of the time.

There are a number of "obstacles" in your way to succeed. Among these are answering questions, finishing in time, and mastering test-taking strategies. All must be executed on the day of the test at peak performance, or your score will suffer. The test is a mental marathon that has a large impact on your future.

Just like a marathon runner, it is important to work your way up to the full challenge. So first you just worry about questions, and then time, and finally strategy:

Success Strategy

1. Find a good source for practice tests.
2. If you are willing to make a larger time investment, consider using more than one study guide- often the different approaches of multiple authors will help you "get" difficult concepts.
3. Take a practice test with no time constraints, with all study helps "open book." Take your time with questions and focus on applying strategies.
4. Take a practice test with time constraints, with all guides "open book."
5. Take a final practice test with no open material and time limits

If you have time to take more practice tests, just repeat step 5. By gradually exposing yourself to the full rigors of the test environment, you will condition your mind to the stress of test day and maximize your success.

Secret Key #4 - **Prepare, Don't Procrastinate**

Let me state an obvious fact: if you take the test three times, you will get three different scores. This is due to the way you feel on test day, the level of preparedness you have, and, despite the test writers' claims to the contrary, some tests WILL be easier for you than others.

Since your future depends so much on your score, you should maximize your chances of success. In order to maximize the likelihood of success, you've got to prepare in advance. This means taking practice tests and spending time learning the information and test taking strategies you will need to succeed.

Never take the test as a "practice" test, expecting that you can just take it again if you need to. Feel free to take sample tests on your own, but when you go to take the official test, be prepared, be focused, and do your best the first time!

Secret Key #5 - Test Yourself

Everyone knows that time is money. There is no need to spend too much of your time or too little of your time preparing for the test. You should only spend as much of your precious time preparing as is necessary for you to get the score you need.

Once you have taken a practice test under real conditions of time constraints, then you will know if you are ready for the test or not.

If you have scored extremely high the first time that you take the practice test, then there is not much point in spending countless hours studying. You are already there.

Benchmark your abilities by retaking practice tests and seeing how much you have improved. Once you score high enough to guarantee success, then you are ready.

If you have scored well below where you need, then knuckle down and begin studying in earnest. Check your improvement regularly through the use of practice tests under real conditions. Above all, don't worry, panic, or give up. The key is perseverance!

Then, when you go to take the test, remain confident and remember how well you did on the practice tests. If you can score high enough on a practice test, then you can do the same on the real thing.

General Strategies

The most important thing you can do is to ignore your fears and jump into the test immediately- do not be overwhelmed by any strange-sounding terms. You have to jump into the test like jumping into a pool- all at once is the easiest way.

Make Predictions

As you read and understand the question, try to guess what the answer will be. Remember that several of the answer choices are wrong, and once you begin reading them, your mind will immediately become cluttered with answer choices designed to throw you off. Your mind is typically the most focused immediately after you have read the question and digested its contents. If you can, try to predict what the correct answer will be. You may be surprised at what you can predict.

Quickly scan the choices and see if your prediction is in the listed answer choices. If it is, then you can be quite confident that you have the right answer. It still won't hurt to check the other answer choices, but most of the time, you've got it!

Answer the Question

It may seem obvious to only pick answer choices that answer the question, but the test writers can create some excellent answer choices that are wrong. Don't pick an answer just because it sounds right, or you believe it to be true. It MUST answer the question. Once you've made your selection, always go back and check it against the question and make sure that you didn't misread the question, and the answer choice does answer the question posed.

Benchmark

After you read the first answer choice, decide if you think it sounds correct or not. If it doesn't, move on to the next answer choice. If it does, mentally mark that answer choice. This doesn't mean that you've definitely selected it as your answer choice, it just means that it's the best you've seen thus far. Go ahead and read the next choice. If the next choice is worse than the one you've already selected, keep going to the next answer choice. If the next choice is better than the choice you've already selected, mentally mark the new answer choice as your best guess.

The first answer choice that you select becomes your standard. Every other answer choice must be benchmarked against that standard. That choice is correct until proven otherwise by another answer choice beating it out. Once you've decided that no other answer choice seems as good, do one final check to ensure that your answer choice answers the question posed.

Valid Information

Don't discount any of the information provided in the question. Every piece of information may be necessary to determine the correct answer. None of the information in the question is there to throw you off (while the answer choices will certainly have information to throw you off). If two seemingly unrelated topics are discussed, don't ignore either. You can be confident there is a relationship, or it wouldn't be included in the question, and you are probably going to have to determine what is that relationship to find the answer.

Avoid "Fact Traps"

Don't get distracted by a choice that is factually true. Your search is for the answer that answers the question. Stay focused and don't fall for an answer that is true but incorrect. Always go back to the question and make sure you're choosing an answer that actually answers the question and is not just a true statement. An answer can be factually correct, but it MUST answer the question asked. Additionally, two answers can both be seemingly correct, so be sure to read all of the answer choices, and make sure that you get the one that BEST answers the question.

Milk the Question

Some of the questions may throw you completely off. They might deal with a subject you have not been exposed to, or one that you haven't reviewed in years. While your lack of knowledge about the subject will be a hindrance, the question itself can give you many clues that will help you find the correct answer. Read the question carefully and look for clues. Watch particularly for adjectives and nouns describing difficult terms or words that you don't recognize. Regardless of if you completely understand a word or not, replacing it with a synonym either provided or one you more familiar with may help you to understand what the questions are asking. Rather than wracking your mind about specific detailed information concerning a difficult term or word, try to use mental substitutes that are easier to understand.

The Trap of Familiarity

Don't just choose a word because you recognize it. On difficult questions, you may not recognize a number of words in the answer choices. The test writers don't put "make-believe" words on the test; so don't think that just because you only recognize all the words in one answer choice means that answer choice must be correct. If you only recognize words in one answer choice, then focus on that one. Is it correct? Try your best to determine if it is correct. If it is, that is great, but if it doesn't, eliminate it. Each word and answer choice you eliminate increases your chances of getting the question correct, even if you then have to guess among the unfamiliar choices.

Eliminate Answers

Eliminate choices as soon as you realize they are wrong. But be careful! Make sure you consider all of the possible answer choices. Just because one appears right, doesn't mean that the next one won't be even better! The test writers will usually put more than one good answer choice for every question, so read all of them. Don't worry if you are stuck between two that seem right. By getting down to just two remaining possible choices, your odds are now 50/50. Rather than wasting too much time, play the odds. You are guessing, but guessing wisely, because you've been able to knock out some of the answer choices that you know are wrong. If you are eliminating choices and realize that the last answer choice you are left with is also obviously wrong, don't panic. Start over and consider each choice again. There may easily be something that you missed the first time and will realize on the second pass.

Tough Questions

If you are stumped on a problem or it appears too hard or too difficult, don't waste time. Move on! Remember though, if you can quickly check for obviously incorrect answer choices, your chances of guessing correctly are greatly improved. Before you completely give up, at least try to knock out a couple of possible answers. Eliminate what you can and then guess at the remaining answer choices before moving on.

Brainstorm

If you get stuck on a difficult question, spend a few seconds quickly brainstorming. Run through the complete list of possible answer choices. Look at each choice and ask yourself, "Could this answer the question satisfactorily?" Go through each answer choice and consider it independently of the other. By systematically going through all possibilities, you may find something that you would otherwise overlook. Remember that when you get stuck, it's important to try to keep moving.

Read Carefully

Understand the problem. Read the question and answer choices carefully. Don't miss the question because you misread the terms. You have plenty of time to read each question thoroughly and make sure you understand what is being asked. Yet a happy medium must be attained, so don't waste too much time. You must read carefully, but efficiently.

Face Value

When in doubt, use common sense. Always accept the situation in the problem at face value. Don't read too much into it. These problems will not require you to make huge leaps of logic. The test writers aren't trying to throw you off with a cheap trick. If you have to go beyond creativity and make a leap of logic in order to have an answer choice answer the question, then you should look at the other answer choices. Don't overcomplicate the problem by creating theoretical relationships or explanations that will warp time or space. These are normal problems rooted in reality. It's just that the applicable relationship or explanation may not be readily apparent and you have to figure things out. Use your common sense to interpret anything that isn't clear.

Prefixes

If you're having trouble with a word in the question or answer choices, try dissecting it. Take advantage of every clue that the word might include. Prefixes and suffixes can be a huge help. Usually they allow you to determine a basic meaning. Pre- means before, post- means after, pro - is positive, de- is negative. From these prefixes and suffixes, you can get an idea of the general meaning of the word and try to put it into context. Beware though of any traps. Just because con is the opposite of pro, doesn't necessarily mean congress is the opposite of progress!

Hedge Phrases

Watch out for critical "hedge" phrases, such as likely, may, can, will often, sometimes, often, almost, mostly, usually, generally, rarely, sometimes. Question writers insert these hedge phrases to cover every possibility. Often an answer choice will be wrong simply because it leaves no room for exception. Avoid answer choices that have definitive words like "exactly," and "always".

Switchback Words

Stay alert for "switchbacks". These are the words and phrases frequently used to alert you to shifts in thought. The most common switchback word is "but". Others include although, however, nevertheless, on the other hand, even though, while, in spite of, despite, regardless of.

New Information

Correct answer choices will rarely have completely new information included. Answer choices typically are straightforward reflections of the material asked about and will directly relate to the question. If a new piece of information is included in an answer choice that doesn't even seem to relate to the topic being asked about, then that answer choice is likely incorrect. All of the information needed to answer the question is usually provided for you, and so you should not have to make guesses that are unsupported or choose answer choices that require unknown information that cannot be reasoned on its own.

Time Management

On technical questions, don't get lost on the technical terms. Don't spend too much time on any one question. If you don't know what a term means, then since you don't have a dictionary, odds are you aren't going to get much further. You should immediately recognize terms as whether or not you know them. If you don't, work with the other clues that you have, the other answer choices and terms provided, but don't waste too much time trying to figure out a difficult term.

Contextual Clues

Look for contextual clues. An answer can be right but not correct. The contextual clues will help you find the answer that is most right and is correct. Understand the context in which a phrase or statement is made. This will help you make important distinctions.

Don't Panic

Panicking will not answer any questions for you. Therefore, it isn't helpful. When you first see the question, if your mind goes blank, take a deep breath. Force yourself to mechanically go through the steps of solving the problem and using the strategies you've learned.

Pace Yourself

Don't get clock fever. It's easy to be overwhelmed when you're looking at a page full of questions, your mind is full of random thoughts and feeling confused, and the clock is ticking down faster than you would like. Calm down and maintain the pace that you have set for yourself. As long as you are on track by monitoring your pace, you are guaranteed to have enough time for yourself. When you get to the last few minutes of the test, it may seem like you won't have enough time left, but if you only have as many questions as you should have left at that point, then you're right on track!

Answer Selection

The best way to pick an answer choice is to eliminate all of those that are wrong, until only one is left and confirm that is the correct answer. Sometimes though, an answer choice may immediately look right. Be careful! Take a second to make sure that the other choices are not equally obvious. Don't make a hasty mistake. There are only two times that you should stop before checking other answers. First is when you are positive that the answer choice you have selected is correct. Second is when time is almost out and you have to make a quick guess!

Check Your Work

Since you will probably not know every term listed and the answer to every question, it is important that you get credit for the ones that you do know. Don't miss any questions through careless mistakes. If at all possible, try to take a second to look back over your answer selection and make sure you've selected the correct answer choice and haven't made a costly careless mistake (such as marking an answer choice that you didn't mean to mark). This quick double check should more than pay for itself in caught mistakes for the time it costs.

Beware of Directly Quoted Answers

Sometimes an answer choice will repeat word for word a portion of the question or reference section. However, beware of such exact duplication – it may be a trap! More than likely, the correct choice will paraphrase or summarize a point, rather than being exactly the same wording.

Slang

Scientific sounding answers are better than slang ones. An answer choice that begins "To compare the outcomes..." is much more likely to be correct than one that begins "Because some people insisted..."

Extreme Statements

Avoid wild answers that throw out highly controversial ideas that are proclaimed as established fact. An answer choice that states the "process should be used in certain situations, if..." is much more likely to be correct than one that states the "process should be discontinued completely."   The first is a calm rational statement and doesn't even make a definitive, uncompromising stance, using a hedge word "if" to provide wiggle room, whereas the second choice is a radical idea and far more extreme.

Answer Choice Families

When you have two or more answer choices that are direct opposites or parallels, one of them is usually the correct answer. For instance, if one answer choice states "x increases" and another answer choice states "x decreases" or "y increases," then those two or three answer choices are very similar in construction and fall into the same family of answer choices. A family of answer choices is when two or three answer choices are very similar in construction, and yet often have a directly opposite meaning. Usually the correct answer choice will be in that family of answer choices. The "odd man out" or answer choice that doesn't seem to fit the parallel construction of the other answer choices is more likely to be incorrect.

Special Report: What Your Test Score Will Tell You About Your IQ

Did you know that most standardized tests correlate very strongly with IQ? In fact, your general intelligence is a better predictor of your success than any other factor, and most tests intentionally measure this trait to some degree to ensure that those selected by the test are truly qualified for the test's purposes.

Before we can delve into the relation between your test score and IQ, I will first have to explain what exactly is IQ. Here's the formula:

Your IQ = 100 + (Number of standard deviations below or above the average)*15

Now, let's define standard deviations by using an example. If we have 5 people with 5 different heights, then first we calculate the average. Let's say the average was 65 inches. The standard deviation is the "average distance" away from the average of each of the members. It is a direct measure of variability - if the 5 people included Jackie Chan and Shaquille O'Neal, obviously there's a lot more variability in that group than a group of 5 sisters who are all within 6 inches in height of each other. The standard deviation uses a number to characterize the average range of difference within a group.

A convenient feature of most groups is that they have a "normal" distribution- makes sense that most things would be normal, right? Without getting into a bunch of statistical mumbo-jumbo, you just need to know that if you know the average of the group and the standard deviation, you can successfully predict someone's percentile rank in the group.

Confused? Let me give you an example. If instead of 5 people's heights, we had 100 people, we could figure out their rank in height JUST by knowing the average, standard deviation, and their height. We wouldn't need to know each person's height and manually rank them, we could just predict their rank based on three numbers.

What this means is that you can take your PERCENTILE rank that is often given with your test and relate this to your RELATIVE IQ of people taking the test - that is, your IQ relative to the people taking the test. Obviously, there's no way to know your actual IQ because the people taking a standardized test are usually not very good samples of the general population- many of those with extremely low IQ's never achieve a level of success or competency necessary to complete a typical standardized test. In fact, professional psychologists who measure IQ actually have to use non-written tests that can fairly measure the IQ of those not able to complete a traditional test.

The bottom line is to not take your test score too seriously, but it is fun to compute your "relative IQ" among the people who took the test with you. I've done the calculations below. Just look up your percentile rank in the left and then you'll see your "relative IQ" for your test in the right hand column-

Percentile Rank	Your Relative IQ		Percentile Rank	Your Relative IQ
99	135		59	103
98	131		58	103
97	128		57	103
96	126		56	102
95	125		55	102
94	123		54	102
93	122		53	101
92	121		52	101
91	120		51	100
90	119		50	100
89	118		49	100
88	118		48	99
87	117		47	99
86	116		46	98
85	116		45	98
84	115		44	98
83	114		43	97
82	114		42	97
81	113		41	97
80	113		40	96
79	112		39	96
78	112		38	95
77	111		37	95
76	111		36	95
75	110		35	94
74	110		34	94
73	109		33	93
72	109		32	93
71	108		31	93
70	108		30	92
69	107		29	92
68	107		28	91
67	107		27	91
66	106		26	90
65	106		25	90
64	105		24	89
63	105		23	89
62	105		22	88
61	104		21	88
60	104		20	87

Special Report: How to Overcome Test Anxiety

The very nature of tests caters to some level of anxiety, nervousness or tension, just as we feel for any important event that occurs in our lives. A little bit of anxiety or nervousness can be a good thing. It helps us with motivation, and makes achievement just that much sweeter. However, too much anxiety can be a problem; especially if it hinders our ability to function and perform.

"Test anxiety," is the term that refers to the emotional reactions that some test-takers experience when faced with a test or exam. Having a fear of testing and exams is based upon a rational fear, since the test-taker's performance can shape the course of an academic career. Nevertheless, experiencing excessive fear of examinations will only interfere with the test-takers ability to perform, and his/her chances to be successful.

There are a large variety of causes that can contribute to the development and sensation of test anxiety. These include, but are not limited to lack of performance and worrying about issues surrounding the test.

Lack of Preparation

Lack of preparation can be identified by the following behaviors or situations:

Not scheduling enough time to study, and therefore cramming the night before the test or exam
Managing time poorly, to create the sensation that there is not enough time to do everything
Failing to organize the text information in advance, so that the study material consists of the entire text and not simply the pertinent information
Poor overall studying habits

Worrying, on the other hand, can be related to both the test taker, or many other factors around him/her that will be affected by the results of the test. These include worrying about:

Previous performances on similar exams, or exams in general
How friends and other students are achieving
The negative consequences that will result from a poor grade or failure

There are three primary elements to test anxiety. Physical components, which involve the same typical bodily reactions as those to acute anxiety (to be discussed below). Emotional factors have to do with fear or panic. Mental or cognitive issues concerning attention spans and memory abilities.

Physical Signals

There are many different symptoms of test anxiety, and these are not limited to mental and emotional strain. Frequently there are a range of physical signals that will let a test taker know that he/she is suffering from test anxiety. These bodily changes can include the following:

Perspiring
Sweaty palms
Wet, trembling hands
Nausea
Dry mouth
A knot in the stomach
Headache
Faintness
Muscle tension
Aching shoulders, back and neck
Rapid heart beat
Feeling too hot/cold

To recognize the sensation of test anxiety, a test-taker should monitor him/herself for the following sensations:

The physical distress symptoms as listed above
Emotional sensitivity, expressing emotional feelings such as the need to cry or laugh too much, or a sensation of anger or helplessness
A decreased ability to think, causing the test-taker to blank out or have racing thoughts that are hard to organize or control.

Though most students will feel some level of anxiety when faced with a test or exam, the majority can cope with that anxiety and maintain it at a manageable level. However, those who cannot are faced with a very real and very serious condition, which can and should be controlled for the immeasurable benefit of this sufferer.

Naturally, these sensations lead to negative results for the testing experience. The most common effects of test anxiety have to do with nervousness and mental blocking.

Nervousness

Nervousness can appear in several different levels:

The test-taker's difficulty, or even inability to read and understand the questions on the test
The difficulty or inability to organize thoughts to a coherent form
The difficulty or inability to recall key words and concepts relating to the testing questions (especially essays)

The receipt of poor grades on a test, though the test material was well known by the test taker

Conversely, a person may also experience mental blocking, which involves:

Blanking out on test questions
Only remembering the correct answers to the questions when the test has already finished.

Fortunately for test anxiety sufferers, beating these feelings, to a large degree, has to do with proper preparation. When a test taker has a feeling of preparedness, then anxiety will be dramatically lessened.

The first step to resolving anxiety issues is to distinguish which of the two types of anxiety are being suffered. If the anxiety is a direct result of a lack of preparation, this should be considered a normal reaction, and the anxiety level (as opposed to the test results) shouldn't be anything to worry about. However, if, when adequately prepared, the test-taker still panics, blanks out, or seems to overreact, this is not a fully rational reaction. While this can be considered normal too, there are many ways to combat and overcome these effects.

Remember that anxiety cannot be entirely eliminated, however, there are ways to minimize it, to make the anxiety easier to manage. Preparation is one of the best ways to minimize test anxiety. Therefore the following techniques are wise in order to best fight off any anxiety that may want to build.

To begin with, try to avoid cramming before a test, whenever it is possible. By trying to memorize an entire term's worth of information in one day, you'll be shocking your system, and not giving yourself a very good chance to absorb the information. This is an easy path to anxiety, so for those who suffer from test anxiety, cramming should not even be considered an option.

Instead of cramming, work throughout the semester to combine all of the material which is presented throughout the semester, and work on it gradually as the course goes by, making sure to master the main concepts first, leaving minor details for a week or so before the test.

To study for the upcoming exam, be sure to pose questions that may be on the examination, to gauge the ability to answer them by integrating the ideas from your texts, notes and lectures, as well as any supplementary readings.

If it is truly impossible to cover all of the information that was covered in that particular term, concentrate on the most important portions, that can be covered very well. Learn these concepts as best as possible, so that when the test comes, a goal can be made to use these concepts as presentations of your knowledge.

In addition to study habits, changes in attitude are critical to beating a struggle with test anxiety. In fact, an improvement of the perspective over the entire test-taking experience can actually help a test taker to enjoy studying and therefore improve the overall experience. Be certain not to overemphasize the significance of the grade - know that the result of the test is neither a reflection of self worth, nor is it a measure of intelligence; one grade will not predict a person's future success.

To improve an overall testing outlook, the following steps should be tried:

Keeping in mind that the most reasonable expectation for taking a test is to expect to try to demonstrate as much of what you know as you possibly can.
Reminding ourselves that a test is only one test; this is not the only one, and there will be others.
The thought of thinking of oneself in an irrational, all-or-nothing term should be avoided at all costs.
A reward should be designated for after the test, so there's something to look forward to. Whether it be going to a movie, going out to eat, or simply visiting friends, schedule it in advance, and do it no matter what result is expected on the exam.

Test-takers should also keep in mind that the basics are some of the most important things, even beyond anti-anxiety techniques and studying. Never neglect the basic social, emotional and biological needs, in order to try to absorb information. In order to best achieve, these three factors must be held as just as important as the studying itself.

Study Steps

Remember the following important steps for studying:

Maintain healthy nutrition and exercise habits. Continue both your recreational activities and social pass times. These both contribute to your physical and emotional well being.
Be certain to get a good amount of sleep, especially the night before the test, because when you're overtired you are not able to perform to the best of your best ability.
Keep the studying pace to a moderate level by taking breaks when they are needed, and varying the work whenever possible, to keep the mind fresh instead of getting bored.
When enough studying has been done that all the material that can be learned has been learned, and the test taker is prepared for the test, stop studying and do something relaxing such as listening to music, watching a movie, or taking a warm bubble bath.

There are also many other techniques to minimize the uneasiness or apprehension that is experienced along with test anxiety before, during, or even after the examination. In fact, there are a great deal of things that can be done to stop anxiety from interfering with lifestyle and performance. Again, remember that anxiety will not be eliminated entirely, and it shouldn't be. Otherwise that "up" feeling for exams would not exist, and most of us depend on that sensation to perform better than usual. However, this anxiety has to be at a level that is manageable.

Of course, as we have just discussed, being prepared for the exam is half the battle right away. Attending all classes, finding out what knowledge will be expected on the exam, and knowing the exam schedules are easy steps to lowering anxiety. Keeping up with work will remove the need to cram, and efficient study habits will eliminate wasted time. Studying should be done in an ideal location for concentration, so that it is simple to become interested in the material and give it complete attention. A method such as SQ3R (Survey, Question, Read, Recite, Review) is a wonderful key to follow to make sure that the study habits are as effective as possible, especially in the case of learning from a textbook. Flashcards are great techniques for memorization. Learning to take good notes will mean that notes will be full of useful information, so that less sifting will need to be done to seek out what is pertinent for studying. Reviewing notes after class and then again on occasion will keep the information fresh in the mind. From notes that have been taken summary sheets and outlines can be made for simpler reviewing.

A study group can also be a very motivational and helpful place to study, as there will be a sharing of ideas, all of the minds can work together, to make sure that everyone understands, and the studying will be made more interesting because it will be a social occasion.

Basically, though, as long as the test-taker remains organized and self confident, with efficient study habits, less time will need to be spent studying, and higher grades will be achieved.

To become self confident, there are many useful steps. The first of these is "self talk." It has been shown through extensive research, that self-talk for students who suffer from test anxiety, should be well monitored, in order to make sure that it contributes to self confidence as opposed to sinking the student. Frequently the self talk of test-anxious students is negative or self-defeating, thinking that everyone else is smarter and faster, that they always mess up, and that if they don't do well, they'll fail the entire course. It is important to decreasing anxiety that awareness is made of self talk. Try writing any negative self thoughts and then disputing them with a positive statement instead. Begin self-encouragement as though it was a friend speaking. Repeat positive statements to help reprogram the mind to believing in successes instead of failures.

Helpful Techniques

Other extremely helpful techniques include:

Self-visualization of doing well and reaching goals
While aiming for an "A" level of understanding, don't try to "overprotect" by setting your expectations lower. This will only convince the mind to stop studying in order to meet the lower expectations.
Don't make comparisons with the results or habits of other students. These are individual factors, and different things work for different people, causing different results.
Strive to become an expert in learning what works well, and what can be done in order to improve. Consider collecting this data in a journal.
Create rewards for after studying instead of doing things before studying that will only turn into avoidance behaviors.
Make a practice of relaxing - by using methods such as progressive relaxation, self-hypnosis, guided imagery, etc - in order to make relaxation an automatic sensation.

Work on creating a state of relaxed concentration so that concentrating will take on the focus of the mind, so that none will be wasted on worrying.
Take good care of the physical self by eating well and getting enough sleep.
Plan in time for exercise and stick to this plan.

Beyond these techniques, there are other methods to be used before, during and after the test that will help the test-taker perform well in addition to overcoming anxiety.

Before the exam comes the academic preparation. This involves establishing a study schedule and beginning at least one week before the actual date of the test. By doing this, the anxiety of not having enough time to study for the test will be automatically eliminated. Moreover, this will make the studying a much more effective experience, ensuring that the learning will be an easier process. This relieves much undue pressure on the test-taker.

Summary sheets, note cards, and flash cards with the main concepts and examples of these main concepts should be prepared in advance of the actual studying time. A topic should never be eliminated from this process. By omitting a topic because it isn't expected to be on the test is only setting up the test-taker for anxiety should it actually appear on the exam. Utilize the course syllabus for laying out the topics that should be studied. Carefully go over the notes that were made in class, paying special attention to any of the issues that the professor took special care to emphasize while lecturing in class. In the textbooks, use the chapter review, or if possible, the chapter tests, to begin your review.

It may even be possible to ask the instructor what information will be covered on the exam, or what the format of the exam will be (for example, multiple choice, essay, free form, true-false). Additionally, see if it is possible to find out how many questions will be on the test. If a review sheet or sample test has been offered by the professor, make good use of it, above anything else, for the preparation for the test. Another great resource for getting to know the examination is reviewing tests from previous semesters. Use these tests to review, and aim to achieve a 100% score on each of the possible topics. With a few exceptions, the goal that you set for yourself is the highest one that you will reach.

Take all of the questions that were assigned as homework, and rework them to any other possible course material. The more problems reworked, the more skill and confidence will form as a result. When forming the solution to a problem, write out each of the steps. Don't simply do head work. By doing as many steps on paper as possible, much clarification and therefore confidence will be formed. Do this with as many homework problems as possible, before checking the answers. By checking the answer after each problem, a reinforcement will exist, that will not be on the exam. Study situations should be as exam-like as possible, to prime the test-taker's system for the experience. By waiting to check the answers at the end, a psychological advantage will be formed, to decrease the stress factor.

Another fantastic reason for not cramming is the avoidance of confusion in concepts, especially when it comes to mathematics. 8-10 hours of study will become one hundred percent more effective if it is spread out over a week or at least several days, instead of doing it all in one sitting. Recognize that the human brain requires time in order to assimilate new material, so frequent breaks and a span of study time over several days will be much more beneficial.

Additionally, don't study right up until the point of the exam. Studying should stop a minimum of one hour before the exam begins. This allows the brain to rest and put things in their proper order. This will also provide the time to become as relaxed as possible when going into the examination room. The test-taker will also have time to eat well and eat sensibly. Know that the brain needs food as much as the rest of the body. With enough food and enough sleep, as well as a relaxed attitude, the body and the mind are primed for success.

Avoid any anxious classmates who are talking about the exam. These students only spread anxiety, and are not worth sharing the anxious sentimentalities.

Before the test also involves creating a positive attitude, so mental preparation should also be a point of concentration. There are many keys to creating a positive attitude. Should fears become rushing in, make a visualization of taking the exam, doing well, and seeing an A written on the paper. Write out a list of affirmations that will bring a feeling of confidence, such as "I am doing well in my English class," "I studied well and know my material," "I enjoy this class." Even if the affirmations aren't believed at first, it sends a positive message to the subconscious which will result in an alteration of the overall belief system, which is the system that creates reality.

If a sensation of panic begins, work with the fear and imagine the very worst! Work through the entire scenario of not passing the test, failing the entire course, and dropping out of school, followed by not getting a job, and pushing a shopping cart through the dark alley where you'll live. This will place things into perspective! Then, practice deep breathing and create a visualization of the opposite situation - achieving an "A" on the exam, passing the entire course, receiving the degree at a graduation ceremony.

On the day of the test, there are many things to be done to ensure the best results, as well as the most calm outlook. The following stages are suggested in order to maximize test-taking potential:

Begin the examination day with a moderate breakfast, and avoid any coffee or beverages with caffeine if the test taker is prone to jitters. Even people who are used to managing caffeine can feel jittery or light-headed when it is taken on a test day.
Attempt to do something that is relaxing before the examination begins. As last minute cramming clouds the mastering of overall concepts, it is better to use this time to create a calming outlook.
Be certain to arrive at the test location well in advance, in order to provide time to select a location that is away from doors, windows and other distractions, as well as giving enough time to relax before the test begins.
Keep away from anxiety generating classmates who will upset the sensation of stability and relaxation that is being attempted before the exam.
Should the waiting period before the exam begins cause anxiety, create a self-distraction by reading a light magazine or something else that is relaxing and simple.

During the exam itself, read the entire exam from beginning to end, and find out how much time should be allotted to each individual problem. Once writing the exam, should more time be taken for a problem, it should be abandoned, in order to begin another problem. If there is time at the end, the unfinished problem can always be returned to and completed.

Read the instructions very carefully - twice - so that unpleasant surprises won't follow during or after the exam has ended.

When writing the exam, pretend that the situation is actually simply the completion of homework within a library, or at home. This will assist in forming a relaxed atmosphere, and will allow the brain extra focus for the complex thinking function.

Begin the exam with all of the questions with which the most confidence is felt. This will build the confidence level regarding the entire exam and will begin a quality momentum. This will also create encouragement for trying the problems where uncertainty resides.

Going with the "gut instinct" is always the way to go when solving a problem. Second guessing should be avoided at all costs. Have confidence in the ability to do well.

For essay questions, create an outline in advance that will keep the mind organized and make certain that all of the points are remembered. For multiple choice, read every answer, even if the correct one has been spotted - a better one may exist.

Continue at a pace that is reasonable and not rushed, in order to be able to work carefully. Provide enough time to go over the answers at the end, to check for small errors that can be corrected.

Should a feeling of panic begin, breathe deeply, and think of the feeling of the body releasing sand through its pores. Visualize a calm, peaceful place, and include all of the sights, sounds and sensations of this image. Continue the deep breathing, and take a few minutes to continue this with closed eyes. When all is well again, return to the test.

If a "blanking" occurs for a certain question, skip it and move on to the next question. There will be time to return to the other question later. Get everything done that can be done, first, to guarantee all the grades that can be compiled, and to build all of the confidence possible. Then return to the weaker questions to build the marks from there.

Remember, one's own reality can be created, so as long as the belief is there, success will follow. And remember: anxiety can happen later, right now, there's an exam to be written!

After the examination is complete, whether there is a feeling for a good grade or a bad grade, don't dwell on the exam, and be certain to follow through on the reward that was promised...and enjoy it! Don't dwell on any mistakes that have been made, as there is nothing that can be done at this point anyway.

Additionally, don't begin to study for the next test right away. Do something relaxing for a while, and let the mind relax and prepare itself to begin absorbing information again.

From the results of the exam - both the grade and the entire experience, be certain to learn from what has gone on. Perfect studying habits and work some more on confidence in order to make the next examination experience even better than the last one.

Learn to avoid places where openings occurred for laziness, procrastination and day dreaming.

Use the time between this exam and the next one to better learn to relax, even learning to relax on cue, so that any anxiety can be controlled during the next exam. Learn how to relax the body. Slouch in your chair if that helps. Tighten and then relax all of the different muscle groups, one group at a time, beginning with the feet and then working all the way up to the neck and face. This will ultimately relax the muscles more than they were to begin with. Learn how to breathe deeply and comfortably, and focus on this breathing going in and out as a relaxing thought. With every exhale, repeat the word "relax."

As common as test anxiety is, it is very possible to overcome it. Make yourself one of the test-takers who overcome this frustrating hindrance.

Special Report: Retaking the Test: What Are Your Chances at Improving Your Score?

After going through the experience of taking a major test, many test takers feel that once is enough. The test usually comes during a period of transition in the test taker's life, and taking the test is only one of a series of important events. With so many distractions and conflicting recommendations, it may be difficult for a test taker to rationally determine whether or not he should retake the test after viewing his scores.

The importance of the test usually only adds to the burden of the retake decision. However, don't be swayed by emotion. There a few simple questions that you can ask yourself to guide you as you try to determine whether a retake would improve your score:

1. What went wrong? Why wasn't your score what you expected?

Can you point to a single factor or problem that you feel caused the low score? Were you sick on test day? Was there an emotional upheaval in your life that caused a distraction? Were you late for the test or not able to use the full time allotment? If you can point to any of these specific, individual problems, then a retake should definitely be considered.

2. Is there enough time to improve?

Many problems that may show up in your score report may take a lot of time for improvement. A deficiency in a particular math skill may require weeks or months of tutoring and studying to improve. If you have enough time to improve an identified weakness, then a retake should definitely be considered.

3. How will additional scores be used? Will a score average, highest score, or most recent score be used?

Different test scores may be handled completely differently. If you've taken the test multiple times, sometimes your highest score is used, sometimes your average score is computed and used, and sometimes your most recent score is used. Make sure you understand what method will be used to evaluate your scores, and use that to help you determine whether a retake should be considered.

4. Are my practice test scores significantly higher than my actual test score?

If you have taken a lot of practice tests and are consistently scoring at a much higher level than your actual test score, then you should consider a retake. However, if you've taken five practice tests and only one of your scores was higher than your actual test score, or if your practice test scores were only slightly higher than your actual test score, then it is unlikely that you will significantly increase your score.

5. Do I need perfect scores or will I be able to live with this score? Will this score still allow me to follow my dreams?

What kind of score is acceptable to you? Is your current score "good enough?" Do you have to have a certain score in order to pursue the future of your dreams? If you won't be happy with your current score, and there's no way that you could live with it, then you should consider a retake. However, don't get your hopes up. If you are looking for significant improvement, that may or may not be possible. But if you won't be happy otherwise, it is at least worth the effort.
Remember that there are other considerations. To achieve your dream, it is likely that your grades may also be taken into account. A great test score is usually not the only thing necessary to succeed. Make sure that you aren't overemphasizing the importance of a high test score.

Furthermore, a retake does not always result in a higher score. Some test takers will score lower on a retake, rather than higher. One study shows that one-fourth of test takers will achieve a significant improvement in test score, while one-sixth of test takers will actually show a decrease. While this shows that most test takers will improve, the majority will only improve their scores a little and a retake may not be worth the test taker's effort.

Finally, if a test is taken only once and is considered in the added context of good grades on the part of a test taker, the person reviewing the grades and scores may be tempted to assume that the test taker just had a bad day while taking the test, and may discount the low test score in favor of the high grades. But if the test is retaken and the scores are approximately the same, then the validity of the low scores are only confirmed. Therefore, a retake could actually hurt a test taker by definitely bracketing a test taker's score ability to a limited range.

Special Report: Additional Bonus Material

Due to our efforts to try to keep this book to a manageable length, we've created a link that will give you access to all of your additional bonus material.

Please visit http://www.mometrix.com/bonus948/cna to access the information.